APHASIOLOGY

Volume 24   Number 2   February 2010

CONTENTS

APHASIOLOGY

SUBSCRIPTION INFORMATION

Subscription rates to Volume 24, 2010 (12 issues) are as follows:

To institutions (full subscription): £1,419.00 (UK);	€1,874.00 (Europe);	$2,354.00 (Rest of the world).
To institutions (online only): £1,349.00 (UK);	€1,780.00 (Europe);	$2,236.00 (Rest of the world).
To individuals: £597.00 (UK);	€789.00 (Europe);	$991.00 (Rest of the world).

Dollar rate applies to all subscribers outside Europe. Euro rates apply to all subscribers in Europe, except the UK and the Republic of Ireland where the pound sterling rate applies. All subscriptions are payable in advance and all rates include postage. Journals are sent by air to the USA, Canada, Mexico, India, Japan and Australasia. Subscriptions are entered on an annual basis, i.e., January to December. Payment may be made by sterling cheque, dollar cheque, euro cheque, international money order, National Giro or credit cards (Amex, Visa, and Mastercard).

An Institutional subscription to the print edition also includes free access to the online edition for any number of concurrent users across a local area network.

Subscriptions purchased at the personal (print only) rate are strictly for personal, non-commercial use only. The reselling of personal subscriptions is strictly prohibited. Personal subcriptions must be purchased with a personal cheque or credit card. Proof of personal status may be requested. For full information please visit the Journal's homepage.

A subscription to the print edition includes free access for any number of concurrent users across a local area network to the online edition, ISSN 1464-5041.

Print subscriptions are also available to individual members of the British Aphasiology Society (BAS), on application to the Society.

Aphasiology now offers an iOpenAccess option for authors. For more information, see: www.tandf.co.uk/journals/iopenaccess.asp

For a complete and up-to-date guide to Taylor & Francis's journals and books publishing programmes, visit the Taylor and Francis website: http://www.tandf.co.uk/

Aphasiology (USPS 001413) is published monthly by Psychology Press, 27 Church Road, Hove, BN3 2FA, UK. The 2010 US Institutional subscription price is $2,354.00. Periodicals Postage Paid at Jamaica, NY 11431, by US Mailing Agent Air Business Ltd, c/o Worldnet Shipping USA Inc., 149-35 177th Street, Jamaica, New York, NY 11434, USA. US Postmaster: Send address changes to *Aphasiology* (PAPH), Air Business Ltd, C/O Worldnet Shipping USA Inc., 149-35 177th Street, Jamaica, New York, NY 11434, USA.

Orders originating in the following territories should be sent direct to the local distributor.

India: Universal Subscription Agency Pvt. Ltd, 101–102 Community Centre, Malviya Nagar Extn, Post Bag No. 8, Saket, New Delhi 110017.

Japan: Kinokuniya Company Ltd, Journal Department, PO Box 55, Chitose, Tokyo 156.

USA, Canada and Mexico: Psychology Press, a member of Taylor & Francis, 325 Chestnut St, Philadelphia, PA 19106, USA

UK and other territories: Psychology Press, c/o T&F Customer Services, Informa UK Ltd, Sheepen Place, Colchester, Essex, CO3 3LP, Tel: +44 (0)20 7017 5544; Fax: +44 (0)20 7017 5198; UK. E-mail: tf.enquiries@tfinforma.com

The online edition can be reached via the journal's website: http://www.psypress.com/aphasiology

Back issues: Taylor & Francis retains a three-year back issue stock of journals. Older volumes are held by our official stockists: Periodicals Service Company, 11 Main Street, Germantown, NY 12526, USA, to whom all orders and enquiries should be addressed. Tel: +1 518 537 4700; Fax: +1 518 537 5899; E-mail: psc@periodicals.com; URL: http://www.periodicals.com/tandf.html

---

Psychology Press makes every effort to ensure the accuracy of all the information (the "Content") contained in its publications. However, Psychology Press and its agents and licensors make no representations or warranties whatsoever as to the accuracy, completeness or suitability for any purpose of the Content and disclaim all such representations and warranties whether express or implied to the maximum extent permitted by law. Any views expressed in the publication are the views of the authors and are not the views of Psychology Press.

Typeset by H. Charlesworth & Co. Ltd., Wakefield, UK.

APHASIOLOGY, 2010, 24 (2), 123–125

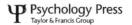

Issues in bilingual aphasia: An introduction

Brendan S. Weekes

University of Sussex, Brighton, UK

At least 50% of the world's population is bilingual and this number is increasing (de Bot, 1992). One important question is how brain damage impacts on the patterns of aphasia observed in the languages of a bilingual speaker. *Language type* constrains these patterns of aphasia (Nilipour & Paradis, 1995). Other constraints are *language status*, i.e., whether a language is acquired first (L1) or acquired later (L2) and *language dominance*, which describes the most familiar language used premorbidly (Paradis, 2008). Variables such as word frequency, imageability, and age of acquisition as well as cognate status—i.e. whether words have similar form and meaning across languages, e.g., blue/bleu in English and French—also impact on patterns of bilingual aphasia.

The aim of this special issue of *Aphasiology* is to examine developments in the study of bilingual aphasia. The extant literature has focused on impressionistic clinical descriptions of bilingual aphasia. However, as case reports become more refined, they have the potential to contribute to development of cognitive models of bilingual language processing. This is the cognitive neuropsychological approach to understanding bilingual language processing (see Beaton & Davies, 2007; Gollan & Kroll, 2001; Weekes & Raman, 2008).

Clinical reports of bilingual aphasia show dissociations in the processing of L1 and L2, with one language more impaired than the other. Other cases show a pattern of differential recovery where L2 is recovered only after L1. Another pattern is alternating antagonism; i.e., patients access one language in spontaneous speech and inhibit the other language for alternating periods (Fabbro, 1999). These patterns raise the question of how the cognitive components of normal bilingual language processing become impaired in aphasia. From a functional perspective this has potential to enhance both assessment and therapy (as in monolingual speakers).

Several papers in this special issue test predictions about preserved and impaired language in bilingual aphasia that are derived from cognitive models of normal bilingual language processing. The paper by Green and colleagues asks whether individuals with bilingual aphasia have difficulties on tasks that require language

Address correspondence to: Department of Psychology, University of Sussex, Falmer, Brighton, BN1 9QG, UK. E-mail: B.S.Weekes@sussex.ac.uk

I would like to acknowledge the support of many colleagues in the preparation of this special issue: Ellen Bialystok, Steven Croft, Wolfgang Dressler, Naama Friedmann, Roel Jonkers, Kathryn Kohnert, Judith Kroll, Sam-Po Law, Jane Marshall, Sara Mondini, Lyndsey Nickels, Ben Parris, Marie-Josephe Tainturier, Ilhan Raman, and Nicole Stadie. Thanks also to Chris Code for supporting this project.

http://www.psypress.com/aphasiology DOI: 10.1080/02687030902958274

control, and show that independent verbal and non-verbal control mechanisms can be selectively impaired. Green et al. also show that impairment to executive processes including the updating of working memory and switching between tasks is relevant to understanding bilingual aphasia. Penn and colleagues continue this theme by reporting that bilingual speakers with aphasia may be less impaired on tasks requiring executive control and show evidence of preserved conversation management. Penn et al. conclude that compensatory behaviours in bilingual aphasia result from enhanced language control compatible with Green's (1998) model. The paper by Hernández and colleagues tests a model of translation by Kroll and Stewart (1994). They report JFF, a premorbidly proficient bilingual with a semantic deficit as a consequence of dementia. JFF's performance suggests the semantic system is involved in both forward (L2→L1) and backward (L1→L2) translation. Hernández and colleagues argue that normal translation performance is a semantic process.

The next section has a focus on the effects of language type in bilingual aphasia; specifically, whether grammatical class effects are different across languages. In the first paper Jarema and colleagues test the hypothesis that morphological distinctions across languages are manifest in bilingual aphasia. They argue that any differences in patterns of aphasia between languages reveal unique properties of the language itself. Jarema et al. show that compound words are represented according to language type. Kambanaros reports that native Greek speakers who acquired English late (after emigration to Australia) produce more verb tokens than noun tokens in conversational speech in contrast to their performance in confrontation naming, showing that language therapy needs to consider word retrieval in non-constrained and constrained contexts. Miozzo and colleagues describe bilingual individuals with selective deficits affecting verb and noun production and the production of irregular and regular verb forms. They conclude that language type has little effect; i.e., grammatical class impairments are similar in bilingual aphasia at least for languages that share morpho-phonological similarities such as Catalan and Spanish.

The remaining papers focus on therapy. Ansaldo and colleagues ask whether L1 or L2 should be used in therapy with bilingual speakers. They argue Green's model offers a rationale for language choice and illustrate this with a Spanish–English bilingual client, EL, who has involuntary language switching. Ansaldo et al. use a self-regulated strategy called *Switch Back Through Translation* to overcome involuntary language switching by translating naming errors into the target language via cueing. Their results reveal evidence of inhibitory mechanisms assumed by Green's model: an internal suppression mechanism allowing translation, and an external suppression mechanism allowing naming. Kiran and Roberts report cross-language and within-language generalisation in three bilingual cases and illustrate how models of normal bilingual language processing can be applied to therapy. Goral and colleagues also examine generalisation after treatment in a trilingual speaker and focus on treatment of morphosyntactic skills. In the treated language, English (L2), there was improvement in production of pronoun gender agreement and this effect generalised to the non-treated language, French (L3), but not to Hebrew (L1). Goral's results suggest that similarities across language type English and French may have more impact than language status; i.e., intervention depends on shared features across language.

REFERENCES

Beaton, A., & Davies, W. (2007). Semantic errors in deep dyslexia: Does orthographic depth matter? *Cognitive Neuropsychology*, *24*(3), 312–323.

de Bot, K. (1992). A bilingual production model: Levelt's 'speaking' model adapted. *Applied Linguistics*, *13*(1), 1–24.

Fabbro, F. (1999). *The neurolinguistics of bilingualism: An introduction*. Hove, UK: Psychology Press.

Gollan, T., & Kroll, J. F. (2001). Bilingual lexical access. In B. Rapp (Ed.), *The handbook of cognitive neuropsychology: What deficits reveal about the human mind* (pp. 321–345). Philadelphia, PA: Psychology Press.

Green, D. W. (1998). Mental control of the bilingual lexico-semantic system. *Bilingualism: Language and Cognition*, *1*, 67–81.

Kroll, J. F., & Stewart, E. (1994). Category interference in translation and picture naming: Evidence for asymmetric connections between bilingual memory representations. *Journal of Memory and Language*, *33*, 149–174.

Nilipour, R., & Paradis, M. (1995). Breakdown of functional categories in three Farsi–English bilingual aphasic patients. In M. Paradis (Ed.), *Aspects of bilingual aphasia* (pp. 123–138). Oxford, UK: Pergamon Press.

Paradis, M. (2008). Language communication disorders in multilinguals. In B. Stemmer & H. Whitaker (Eds.), *Handbook of the neuroscience of language* (Section V:2). Amsterdam: Elsevier.

Weekes, B. S., & Raman, I. (2008). Bilingual deep dysphasia. *Cognitive Neuropsychology*, *25*(3), 411–436.

APHASIOLOGY, 2010, 24 (2), 126–140

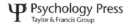

The processing of compounds in bilingual aphasia: A multiple-case study

Gonia Jarema and Danuta Perlak

University of Montreal, and Institut universitaire de gériatrie de Montréal, Montreal, Canada

Carlo Semenza

University of Padova, and I.R.C.C.S. Ospedale S.Camillo, Lido di Venezia, Italy

Background: While converging evidence has led to the view that people with aphasia exploit compositional procedures when producing compound words, the issue of what compound-internal characteristics are at play during these procedures is still under debate. It has been argued that constituent position and/or morphosyntactic prominence, i.e., being the head constituent of a compound, may influence the manner in which compounds are accessed. However, findings obtained from patient performances are thus far inconclusive, because positional and headedness effects are frequently confounded in a language.

Aims: In order to disentangle position-in-the-string and headedness effects in compound production in aphasia, the main objective of this study is to investigate the performance of bilingual patients speaking languages in which these effects can be teased apart. Our secondary goal is to probe the roles of grammatical category (adjectives vs nouns) and of between-language phonological similarity, as both these factors have been demonstrated to influence compound processing.

Methods & Procedures: Three English–French bilingual persons with aphasia participated in the study. Three experimental tasks, reading, repetition, and translation of isolated compound words, were administrated in each language. We contrasted French and English compounds that differ in the position of the head constituent: left for French and right for English.

Outcomes & Results: Two participants showed a similar pattern—a significantly reduced number of errors for the head (or first) constituent as compared to the non-head (or second) constituent in French and an equivalent number of errors for both constituents in English—pointing to the cumulative effects of headedness and first-position-in-the-string in French, and to the mutual cancelling out of these effects in English. The third participant exhibited a non-head constituent advantage in both languages, indicating that semantic modification of the head constituent by the non-head constituent plays a prominent role in her accessing procedures. For all three participants phonological similarity influenced production, while grammatical category did not.

Address correspondence to: Gonia Jarema, Research Centre, Institut universitaire de gériatrie de Montréal, 4565 chemin Queen-Mary, Montreal, Quebec, Canada H3W 1W5.
E-mail: gonia.jarema@umontreal.ca

This research was supported by an MCRI (Major Collaborative Research Initiative) grant (412-2001-1009) from the Social Sciences and Humanities Research Council of Canada. We would like to express special thanks to Fanny Singer, speech therapist and Director of the Department of Speech Therapy at the Jewish Rehabilitation Centre in Laval. We are most grateful to participants RS, GK, and VR for kindly agreeing to participate in this study.

http://www.psypress.com/aphasiology   DOI: 10.1080/02687030902958225

Conclusions: Our results reveal that headedness and position *interact* in the processing of compounds. They also demonstrate that compound constituents are processed asymmetrically across and within languages, thus confirming that people with aphasia are sensitive to compound-internal structure. Moreover, they show that patients rely on varying structural information when accessing compounds.

Keywords: Bilingual aphasia; Compound processing; Headedness; Position-in-the-string; Semantic modification.

Central to the cognitive system subserving language is the ability to create new words. One of the most universal and productive lexical devices for expanding a language's vocabulary is that of compounding, a mechanism by which novel words are created by conjoining existing words. Compounds are thus complex, or polymorphemic, lexical entities (e.g., the words *blueberry* and *tablecloth* each contain two subcomponents, or morphemes) and as such may present a particular challenge to individuals with impaired linguistic abilities. Studies conducted in a variety of tasks and in a variety of languages have shown that compounds can be named, repeated, read, and written erroneously by people with aphasia, and recurring patterns of breakdown in their performances have led to important insights into the processing of compounds in aphasia. These include the observation that people with aphasia seem to be cognisant, whether implicitly or explicitly, of compound-internal structure (Badecker, 2001; Blanken, 2000; Delazer & Semenza, 1998; Hittmair-Delazer, Andrée, Semenza, De Bleser, & Benke, 1994; Mäkisalo, Niemi, & Laine, 1999), indicating in turn that compounds are not solely accessed as whole-word units, or "chunks". Constituent structure is clearly at play during compound processing, because patients tend to substitute (Badecker, 2001; Blanken, 2000; Delazer & Semenza, 1998; Mäkisalo et al., 1999) and omit (Blanken, 2000; Delazer & Semenza, 1998; Hittmair-Delazer et al., 1994) only one of the compound's constituents in spontaneous speech and when performing various production tasks. This had led to the claim that the internal structure of a compound is exploited during lexical access and that compound processing is compositional (for an extensive discussion of a compositional account of compound production, see Badecker, 2001).

While compositional processes appear to be well documented, the issue of what structural properties of compounds influence accessing procedures in the performance of people with aphasia remains controversial. One unresolved question concerns the role that "position-in-the-string" may play during compound processing, i.e., whether it is the first or the second constituent of a compound that is more vulnerable to impairment. Investigations conducted over the last decade have yielded inconclusive results. Thus, while awareness of the structural frame of compounds was generally found to be preserved, positional effects varied greatly across studies. For example, in a group study of 15 German-speaking persons with aphasia, Hittmair-Delazer et al. (1994) observed that patients deleted and omitted mostly the first compound constituent in a naming task. A similar finding was reported by Stark and Stark (1990) who found that, in repetition, their German-speaking Wernicke's patient frequently omitted the first constituent of twin compounds (*Orangensaft*, "orange juice", *Saftorangen*, "juice oranges"). By contrast, in a single-case study of an Italian-speaking individual presenting with amnesic aphasia, Delazer and Semenza (1998) reported a total absence of positional effects in the constituent substitutions observed in confrontation naming and naming on description. Interestingly, their patient respected the position of the preserved constituent, which brought to light awareness of compound-internal structure. A somewhat more mixed picture is presented by Blanken (2000) in a group study of German-speaking individuals with aphasia. While across a variety of tasks participants showed no positional effects in their substitution errors, they exhibited a significant second-constituent advantage in their constituent omissions. In their attempts at naming compounds, they also tended to produce the second constituent first.

A further issue under debate is that of the role of 'headedness" in the processing of compounds. In the example *blueberry* cited above, *berry* is the compound's morphosyntactic head. It determines the grammatical category and morphological properties of the compound as a whole. Thus *blueberry* is a noun because the head constituent *berry* is a noun (while *blue* is an adjective). The German compound *Tischdecke* ("tablecloth") is a feminine noun because *Decke* is feminine (while *Tisch* is masculine). The question arises, therefore, whether the privileged status of the head constituent influences processing and determines behavioural patterns in language breakdown. Blanken (2000) related his finding that second-constituent omissions were more frequent than first-constituent omissions to the fact that compounds are right-headed in German. However, as indicated above, Blanken's finding contrasts with that of Stark and Stark (1990) and Hittmai-Delazer et al. (1994), who found a first-constituent, i.e., non-head, advantage for German. Moreover, in the study by Blanken (2000), a headedness effect was obtained only when patients omitted constituents. It was absent in the case of constituent substitutions (the most frequent error type), which were equally distributed between first (non-head) and second (head) constituents. Yet other studies found no headedness effect at all (e.g., Delazer & Semenza, 1998).

As is evident from the studies reviewed above, a major problem underlying efforts to understand the respective roles of constituent position and headedness in the processing of compounds is the fact that in languages such as English or German, i.e., languages in which the head is always in second position, positional and headedness effects cannot be easily teased apart. One approach to resolving the problem might be to contrast left- and right-headed compounds within one and the same language (in languages that feature left- and right-headed compounds) or across languages. This is precisely what Jarema, Busson, Nikolova, Tsapkini, and Libben (1999) undertook to do in a combined within-language and cross-language investigation comparing French (in which compounds can be left- *or* right-headed) and Bulgarian (in which compounds are always right-headed, as in English or German) in the performance of unimpaired individuals on a primed lexical decision task. The study revealed that French-speaking participants showed a significant left-constituent advantage for left-headed compounds, e.g., *garçon manqué* (lit. boy failed, "tomboy"). By contrast, a greater magnitude of priming was not obtained for second-constituent primes as compared to first-constituent primes in the case of right-headed compounds, e.g., *grasse matiné* (lit. fat morning, "sleep-in"). Bulgarian, on the other hand, did not yield differential priming patterns. Taken together, these findings reveal that position-in-the-string and headedness interact in compound processing across languages.

To date, the problem of disentangling the effects of position-in-the-string vs headedness in the processing of compounds has, to our knowledge, not been directly addressed in the aphasiological literature. The main objective of the present study is therefore to investigate this issue in the performance of bilingual language-impaired individuals who are speakers of languages that contrast with regard to the position of the head of compounds. We hypothesise that if position-in-the-string and headedness do play a critical role in the processing of compounds, these effects should emerge differentially across the two languages. We tested bilinguals rather than monolinguals in an effort to circumvent the confound of inter-participant variability. Factors such as age, sex, level of education, lesion site, aphasia type, and degree of severity are difficult to hold constant when contrasting two languages across monolingual patients. Bilingual patients, on the other hand, may be considered as their own controls. The following experiment presents results from the performances of English–French bilingual persons with aphasia tested on their ability to produce right-headed English and left-headed French compounds.

METHOD

Participants

Three persons with aphasia participated in this study. RS was a 75-year-old right-handed man with 15 years of education, who had worked as a financial planner and headed his own company. He suffered a stroke in August 1998, 8 years prior to the onset of this investigation; his CT scan indicated damage to the left frontoparietal area. Medical examination revealed full ocular movement; upper and lower extremity strength was intact and fine coordinate movement was adequately performed; muscle testing evidenced mild right-sided weakness of labial and lingual muscles. RS was diagnosed with mild-to-moderate non-fluent aphasia using the Minnesota Test for Differential Diagnosis of Aphasia (Schuell & Sefer, 1973). His auditory comprehension was found to be mildly impaired, while verbal expression and reading comprehension were moderately impaired. Written expression was moderately impaired at the sentence level, with dysgraphia. RS returned to work in January 1999.

GK was a 60-year-old right-handed man with 15 years of education and holding a certificate in accounting. He worked in the finance department of a leasing company, of which he was the vice-president. Prior to that he had worked in a bank for 10 years. GK's cerebro-vascular accident occurred in January 2000, 6 years before he participated in this study; an angiogram demonstrated a ruptured left middle cerebral artery aneurysm; his CT scan showed a perfusion in the left basal cisterns, as well as in the anterior fissure and into the left basal Sylvian fissure. GK was left with some right-sided weakness of the arm and leg, which slowly improved. He was diagnosed with severe mixed aphasia using the Minnesota Test for Differential Diagnosis of Aphasia (Schuell & Sefer, 1973). At the end of his therapy in 2000 his auditory comprehension was mildly impaired, verbal expression was severely impaired, reading comprehension was moderately impaired, and written expression was moderately to severely impaired. GK continues to work in banking as a counsellor and manages most of his family's affairs.

VR was a 64-year-old right-handed woman with 15 years of education who worked as a secretary in a primary school. She suffered a thrombotic cerebro-vascular accident in the region of the left middle cerebral artery in July 2006, 9 months prior to the onset of this investigation. She was diagnosed with mild to moderate transcortical sensory aphasia using the Montreal-Toulouse aphasia battery

(Lecours et al., 1986), supplemented by parts of the French version (Mazaux & Orgogozo, 1982) of the BDAE (Boston Diagnostic Aphasia Examination; Kaplan & Goodglass, 1983), including the Token Test. Her auditory comprehension was mildly impaired; written expression, reading comprehension, and verbal expression were mildly to moderately impaired. Verbal expression was characterised by qualitative and quantitative moderate speech reduction and preserved repetition. She also presented moderate dyslexia with preserved access to words and moderate dysorthography.

Three measures were used to develop a language profile of the participants' knowledge of French and English. *Language history* data were collected from responses to three sections of the BAT (Bilingual Aphasia Test; Paradis, 1987): History of Bilingualism, French Background and English Background. The History of Bilingualism subset of the BAT consists of questions about the use of each language in childhood, parental language use patterns, educational experience, and occupational experience. The French Background and English Background subsets include a series of questions specific to each language: age of acquisition, language use at home and at work, and frequency of use. Table 1 summarises the language profiles of the three participants.

Note that the demographics of Montreal (the bilingual city in which all three participants grew up and still live) are such that many people are exposed to a third language in their early childhood, i.e., to the language of first or second generation immigrant family members. Moreover, by virtue of living in a bilingual environment, children from all cultural backgrounds are exposed early on to both French and English, go to French or English schools, and not uncommonly switch from one system to the other. They also learn French or English as a second language from elementary school onwards. They thus grow up in a multicultural environment, where bilingualism coexists with multilingualism. In the case of our participants, SR first learned to speak English and Yiddish, and GK English and Greek. They started learning French at school (at age 6), were partly educated in French and considered themselves fluent in the language. They used both English and French at work and with friends. VR had a francophone mother and spoke French during her early childhood, although her father was Greek. Like SR and GK she had been educated in English for many years and spoke both languages at work. The linguistic backgrounds of SR, GK, and VR thus present several commonalities: all three had

TABLE 1
Language profiles

	RS	*GK*	*VR*
Languages			
Before school age	English & Yiddish	English & Greek	French
Used at work	English & French	English & French	French & English
Spoken pre- and post-onset	English, French & Yiddish	English, French & Greek	French & English
Language of speech therapy	English	English	French
Education			
English	7 years	14 years	7 years
French	8 years	1 year	9 years

some exposure to a third language in their early childhood, were educated in both English and French, and used both languages at work and socially.

In addition, the participants' performances in the two languages were compared using the short version of the BAT (French–English) with each participant. In part B of the BAT, participants RS and GK performed better in English than in French (66% and 76% for RS, 68% and 90% for GK in French and in English, respectively). Paired t-tests indicated that the difference was statistically significant ($t = -2.227$, $p = .04$ for RS and $t = -4.941$, $p = .0008$ for GK) but this is less salient for RS than for GK. Participant VR showed a similar performance in the two languages, 82% of correct responses in French and 78% in English ($t = .700$, $p = .494$). Tables 2 and 3 (see later) show the scores of correct responses in both languages for parts B and C of the BAT for each of the three participants. VR was thus a relatively balanced bilingual, while RS and particularly GK were English dominant.

Stimuli

A list of 80 word pairs was created, comprising 80 French left-headed compounds and 80 English right-headed compounds. In order to control for orthographical/phonological similarity between corresponding French–English compounds, it was decided to test cognates which, by definition, feature maximal formal similarity across languages. In the psycholinguistic (e.g., Costa, Caramazza, & Sebastiàn-Gallés, 2000; de Bot, Cox, Ralston, Schaufeli, & Weltens, 1995; de Groot, Borgwaldt, Bos, & van den Eijinden, 2002) and neuropsychological (e.g., Kohnert, 2004; Lalor & Kirsner, 2001; Roberts & Deslauriers, 1999) literature, cognates (e.g., *liste civile/civil list*) have been found to be more easily accessible and less frequently impaired than non-cognates (e.g., *maître nageur/swimming teacher*). It was therefore decided to further add non-cognate French and English compounds to our stimulus list, in order to also contrast the cognate/non-cognate dimension. For each language, the list thus comprised 30 cognate compounds (noun-adjective in French and adjective-noun in English, e.g., *certificat médical/medical certificate*),[1] 30 non-cognate compounds (noun-adjective in French and adjective-noun in English, e.g., *feuille morte/dead leaf*), and 20 noun-noun compounds (e.g., *café filtre/filter coffee*). Noun-noun compounds were added to the list in order to test the effects of grammatical category within each constituent position, as grammatical category has been found to influence lexical processing (e.g., Mondini, Luzzatti, Zonca, Pistarini, & Semenza, 2004; Semenza, Luzzatti, & Carabelli, 1997). Due to limitations in the availability of comparable stimulus pairs, the group of 30 non-cognate compounds comprised two sub-groups: 12 non-cognate compounds (in which both constituents were non-cognates, e.g., *feuille morte/dead leaf*) and 18 semi-cognate compounds (10 semi-cognate compounds yielding French–English pairs with non-cognate – cognate/cognate – non-cognate constituent structures, e.g., *eau minérale/mineral water*, and 8

---

[1] N–N compounds being much less prevalent in English than in French, an adequate stimulus list of cognate French and English N–N compounds could not be constructed. Instead we used attested French N–A and English A–N compounds that can be distinguished from syntactic phrases by a number of criteria, including the generally accepted criterion of integrity, according to which a compound's constituents cannot be separated by other words or phrases (for a thorough discussion of compound types and criteria put forth to distinguish compounds from other types of phrasal units, see Dressler, 2006, and Spencer, 1991).

TABLE 2
Number of errors in each language and task for each participant

	QRS	GK	VR
FRENCH			
Reading	50	16	20
Repetition	9	14	2
Translation	87	71	38
Total	*146*	*101*	*60*
ENGLISH			
Reading	6	3	26
Repetition	1	3	3
Translation	64	34	58
Total	*71*	*40*	*87*

semi-cognate compounds yielding French–English pairs with cognate – non-cognate/ non-cognate – cognate constituent structures, e.g., *angle droit/right angle*).

In addition, in each language 80 polymorphemic words, matched for letter length and frequency to each particular compound word, were added as distractors. The mean letter length of compound words in French was 12.5 ($SD = 2.7$), and the mean frequency was 0.2 ($SD = 1.8$); for distractor words, the mean letter length was 12.5 ($SD = 2.6$) and the mean frequency was 0.2 ($SD = 1.9$). In English, the mean letter length of compound words was 11.2 ($SD = 2.3$), and the mean frequency was 0 ($SD = 0.2$); for distractor words, the mean letter length was 11.2 ($SD = 2.3$) and the mean frequency was 0 ($SD = 0.2$). We used the BRULEX database (Content, Mousty, & Radeau, 1990) for French and the CELEX database (Baayen, Piepenbrock, & Gulikers, 1995) for English.

Procedure

All participants completed six experimental tasks over several testing sessions. The total number of sessions varied as a function of the individual's speed and frequency of breaks: VR was tested in six 1-hour sessions, RS in eight 1-hour sessions, and GK in ten 1-hour (or more) sessions. Each participant performed three experimental tasks in both French and English: reading, repetition, and translation of a list of words. The tasks were executed in the same order for all participants: reading in French, repetition in English, translation from French to English, reading in English, repetition in French, translation from English to French. In the case of the translation tasks, translation of distractor words from the experimental list was avoided because of the participants' difficulty in translating these items (distractors were matched to compounds and were thus very long and infrequent polymorphemic words).

RESULTS

Error type

In general, errors consisted of phonemic paraphasias, morphological paraphasias, semantic paraphasias, verbal paraphasias, neologisms, deletions of the first or second constituent, constituent inversions, and insertions of a preposition and/or a determiner (in French only, where such constructions are prevalent, e.g., *chasse-à-l'homme*, lit.

hunt-for-the-man, "manhunt"). Overall, in the reading and repetition tasks the most frequent errors were phonemic and morphological paraphasias, while in the translation tasks all types of errors were observed (for examples, see Appendix 1). This latter observation underscores the increased difficulty of translation over reading and repetition for all three participants, as revealed by the following analysis.

Comparing performances between and within tasks

Overall, RS showed a higher number of errors in French than in English ($\chi^2 = 68.25$, $p < .001$): in reading ($\chi^2 = 47.43$, $p < .001$), in repetition ($\chi^2 = 6.83$, $p = .009$), and in translation ($\chi^2 = 48.13$, $p < .001$). He performed better in repetition than in reading in French ($\chi^2 = 45.14$, $p < .001$), while no difference between these two tasks was found in English ($\chi^2 = 2.401$, $p = .117$); his performance in reading and in repetition was better than in translation, and that was the case in both languages ($\chi^2 = 36.92$, $p < .001$; $\chi^2 = 127.64$, $p < .001$ for French, and $\chi^2 = 85.44$, $p < .001$; $\chi^2 = 102.84$, $p < .001$ for English) (see Appendix 2 for number of errors per error type in each language).

As demonstrated for RS, GK showed a higher number of errors in French than in English ($\chi^2 = 51.96$, $p < .001$): in reading ($\chi^2 = 14.15$, $p < .001$), in repetition ($\chi^2 = 10.0$, $p < .002$), and in translation ($\chi^2 = 44.21$, $p < .001$). GK performed similarly well in reading and in repetition in both languages ($\chi^2 = 0.042$, $p = .837$ for French, and $\chi^2 = 1.03$, $p = .311$ for English). Translation was more difficult than reading and repetition in both languages ($\chi^2 = 75.92$, $p < .001$, $\chi^2 = 78.60$, $p < .001$ for French, and $\chi^2 = 26.45$, $p < .001$, $\chi^2 = 20.95$, $p < .001$ for English) (see Appendix 3 for number of errors per error type in each language).

By contrast, VR showed a higher number of errors in English than in French ($\chi^2 = 33.43$, $p < .001$), but the difference was significant only in the translation task ($\chi^2 = 13.58$, $p < .001$), while in reading and in repetition the number of errors did not differ ($\chi^2 = 1.48$, $p = .224$; $\chi^2 = 0.206$, $p = .65$ in reading and in repetition, respectively). In both languages she performed better in repetition than in reading ($\chi^2 = 17.08$, $p < .001$, $\chi^2 = 48.37$, $p < .001$ for French and English, respectively). Her performance in reading and in repetition was better than in translation in both languages ($\chi^2 = 11.68$, $p < .001$, $\chi^2 = 48.37$, $p < .001$ for French, and $\chi^2 = 23.63$, $p < .001$ $\chi^2 = 25.75$, $p < .001$ for English) (see Appendix 4 for number of errors per error type in each language). Table 2 presents the number of errors on each task for each participant.

For all three participants, paired t-tests run in order to compare their performances across the translation tasks (from French to English and from English to French) did not show any significant differences between the two translation directions ($t = -1.213$, $p = .312$; $t = -0.104$, $p = .923$; $t = 1.0$, $p = .391$, for RS, GK, and VR, respectively).

Headedness

Statistics based on an error rate analysis over all tasks and all critical stimuli revealed that RS and GK made significantly fewer errors on the head constituent (C_{head}) than on the non-head constituent ($C_{non-head}$) in French ($\chi^2 = 4.10$, $p = .043$; $\chi^2 = 19.75$, $p < .001$ for RS and GK, respectively) while in English both participants made an equivalent number of errors on the two constituents ($\chi^2 = 0.37$, $p = .543$; $\chi^2 = .046$,

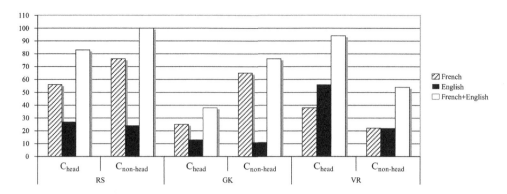

Figure 1. Number of errors on head constituents (C_{head}) and non-head constituents ($C_{non-head}$) for each participant.

$p = .831$ for RS and GK, respectively). In contrast, VR made significantly more errors on C_{head} than on $C_{non-head}$ in French and in English ($\chi^2 = 7.19$, $p < .007$; $\chi^2 = 8.02$, $p < .005$ for French and English, respectively). Differential constituent effects were thus obtained for VR vs RS and GK, pointing to the coming into play of varying accessing mechanisms across the productions of compounds of people with aphasia (see Figure 1).

Phonological/orthographical similarity: Cognates versus non-cognates

For all three participants, performance on semi-cognate compounds with a cognate head did not differ from semi-cognate compounds with a cognate non-head ($\chi^2 = 1.14$, $p = .713$; $\chi^2 = 0.844$, $p = .358$; $\chi^2 = 0.583$, $p = .445$ in French for RS, GK, and VR, respectively, and $\chi^2 = 0.048$, $p = .826$; $\chi^2 = 3.46$, $p = .087$; $\chi^2 = 0.254$, $p = .614$ in English for RS, GK, and VR, respectively). In the case of RS and VR, semi-cognate compounds in French and in English were similar to non-cognate compounds ($\chi^2 = 0.004$, $p = .951$; $\chi^2 = 0.698$, $p = .403$ for RS and VR respectively) and thus the two types of semi-cognate compounds were collapsed. For RS and VR, the comparison between cognate and non-cognate compounds showed that the number of errors did not differ (but approached significance) when comparing cognate and non-cognate compounds in French ($\chi^2 = 3.30$, $p = .069$; $\chi^2 = 3.34$, $p = .068$ for RS and VR, respectively). In English, the number of errors was significantly smaller in the case of cognate compounds as compared to the non-cognate compounds ($\chi^2 = 5.75$, $p = .016$; $\chi^2 = 8.24$, $p = .004$ for RS and VR, respectively), and the same pattern as in English was found in the two languages taken together ($\chi^2 = 7.25$, $p = .007$; $\chi^2 = 11.14$, $p < .001$ for RS and VR, respectively). In the case of GK the statistical analysis demonstrated that semi-cognate compounds were more similar to cognate compounds than to non-cognate compounds ($\chi^2 = 2.86$, $p = .091$). For GK, the semi-cognate compounds were thus included in the group of cognate compounds and the comparison between cognate and non-cognate compounds showed, as it had shown for RS and VR, a smaller number of errors in the case of cognate compounds as compared to non-cognate compounds in both French ($\chi^2 = 17.94$, $p < .001$) and English ($\chi^2 = 11.10$, $p < .001$). These results thus replicate the finding that cognates facilitate lexical processing (Kohnert, 2004; Lalor & Kirsner, 2001; Roberts & Deslauriers, 1999).

Grammatical category: Adjectives vs nouns

Comparing the grammatical category of compound constituents in the same position in the string (right in French N-A vs N-N compounds; left in English A-N vs N-N compounds), an error rate analysis showed no difference between adjective and noun constituents of compounds for RS and GK in French ($\chi^2 = 1.24$, $p = .265$; $\chi^2 = 0.001$, $p = 1.0$ for RS and GK respectively), while VR made more errors on the nominal constituents ($\chi^2 = 5.506$, $p = .027$). For all three participants, no effect of grammatical category was observed in English ($\chi^2 = 0.676$, $p = .796$; $\chi^2 = 2.572$, $p = .149$; $\chi^2 = 0.346$, $p = .556$ for RS, GK and VR, respectively). Thus, overall, adjectives and nouns do not appear to dissociate in the processing of compounds in the performances of RS, GK, and VR, in contrast to findings obtained for verb-noun compounds (e.g., Mondini et al., 2004; Semenza et al., 1997).

DISCUSSION

Using a multiple single-case paradigm, this study aimed at isolating the role of headedness in the processing of compounds by language-impaired individuals. Previous studies reporting positional and headedness effects yielded varying findings and have thus far failed to unambiguously disentangle the relative roles of position-in-the-string and headedness in compound processing in aphasia. The approach adopted in the present study consisted in eliciting the production of French left-headed and English right-headed compounds from persons with aphasia who could be considered as their own controls, i.e., English–French bilinguals. Results from the performances of two of the three participants (SR and GK) offer support for the view that position-in-the-string *and* headedness play a role in compound processing in aphasia, in line with previous findings obtained with language-unimpaired individuals (Jarema et al., 1999). These two participants showed a similar pattern across tasks.[2] French left-headed compounds yielded a significant left-constituent advantage in the number of errors produced, while for English right-headed compounds errors were equally distributed across first and second constituents. Taken together, these results clearly point to an interaction between position-in-the-string and headedness. If headedness alone were at play, then a headedness effect should have been obtained not only for French but also for English, which was not the case. If, on the other hand, position-in-the-string alone played a role, then the first or the second constituent should have shown an advantage in both languages, independently of headedness, which was also not the case. Following Jarema et al.'s (1999) reasoning we thus propose that, in French, the left-constituent advantage can be attributed to the cumulative effects of first position-in-the-string and headedness, while in English the lack of any advantage reflects the mutual cancelling out of these effects.

---

[2] Crucially, this was the case despite the fact that GK had only 1 year of education in French vs 8 for SR, indicating clearly that GK's limited schooling in French did not play a significant role in the effects obtained.

However, the results obtained from our third participant (VR) are puzzling. In her case, the non-head constituent yielded significantly fewer errors than the head constituent and, importantly, this was true of both languages. Thus the right constituent was more vulnerable in French, while the left constituent was more vulnerable in English, indicating that the results obtained could not be reducible to a positional effect. In the absence of either a position-in-the-string or a headedness effect in this participant's production of French and English compounds, what could underlie the stability of the non-head constituent in her performance? An answer can be found in considering the role that this constituent plays within the compound structure. In an adjective-noun compound such as *blueberry*, the non-head constituent *blue* modifies the head constituent. It specifies the type of berry a blueberry is, and thus contributes to distinguishing the meaning of *blueberry* from the meaning of, e.g., *blackberry* or *strawberry*. Similarly, in a noun-noun compound such as *tablecloth*, the non-head constituent *table* modifies the head constituent *cloth*. Modifiers thus play a crucial role in specifying the meaning of compounds, as can be more compellingly illustrated in considering the compound *hotdog*. It can undoubtedly be said that there is very little of a dog in a hotdog—i.e., hardly any features generally associated with the concept of a dog (domestic animal, four-legged, furry, etc.) can be found in *hotdog*. The burden of specifying the idiosyncratic meaning of the compound falls on the modifier *hot*. It alone determines that a hotdog is not a kind of dog while, by contrast, the modifier *lap* in the compound *lapdog* determines that a lapdog *is* a kind of dog—for an extended discussion of the role of modifiers, see Gagné and Spalding (2006) who adopt a relation-based approach to compound processing, in keeping with the Competition-Among-Relations-in-Nominals (CARIN) model proposed by Gagné (2001) and Gagné and Shoben (1997) to account for conceptual combination. We would like to suggest that, for VR, the primacy of the modifying constituent of a compound is of particular salience, resulting in the increased stability of the non-head constituent in her productions of both French and English compounds.

Ultimately, the contrasting pattern obtained with regard to the stability of constituents for RS and GK vs VR points to the well-established inter-participant variability in the performance of persons with aphasia. This variability reflects, among other things, patients' varying residual capacities and varying reliability on specific linguistic properties. Reliance on local morphosyntactic and positional properties seems to dominate in RS and GK's performances, while VR appears to rely mainly on a semantic property of compound formation, i.e., the dominant status of the modifier's semantics in relation to the more general semantics of the "modifyee". This can be conceptualised as an implicit strategy that reflects the relative strengths of available information and the system's capacity to maximise computational efficiency in the presence of increased processing load due to brain damage, by recruiting the most salient linguistic features available. The data presented here offer compelling evidence that both morphological constituency information and semantic modification information are at play during compound processing in aphasia and may be recruited differentially, leading to performance asymmetries among patients. The asymmetry observed in the productions of our participants may reflect differences in aphasia type, with RS's non-fluent and GK's mixed aphasias patterning together and inducing increased sensitivity to one kind of information, and VR's transcortical motor aphasia inducing sensitivity to another kind.

At a more general level, what comes to light in the above is that, in their processing of compounds, all three participants are sensitive to the principle of compositionality. If this were not the case, one would be unable to account for the differential effects obtained across compound constituents. In keeping with previous studies (Badecker, 2001; Blanken, 2000; Delazer & Semenza, 1998; Hittmair-Delazer et al., 1994; Mäkisalo et al., 1999), this systematic intra-compound variation thus clearly demonstrates that constituent activation is involved during the production of compounds in aphasia. The surfacing of compositional effects in this and earlier neuropsychological studies further confirms the structured nature of compound representation and processing advocated in the psycholinguistic literature (e.g., Libben & Jarema, 2006), indicating that similar principles govern compound production in language-impaired and intact populations.

A secondary question addressed in this investigation was whether facilitatory effects previously observed in the processing of cognates vs non-cognates would be replicated in our participants' processing of compounds. Results clearly point to the greater preservation of cognates over non-cognates, thus confirming previous findings obtained from intact (e.g., Costa et al., 2000; de Bot et al., 1995; de Groot et al., 2002) and brain-damaged (e.g., Kohnert, 2004; Lalor & Kirsner, 2001; Roberts & Deslauriers, 1999) populations.

Prompted by previous findings that grammatical category influences lexical processing in aphasia (Mondini et al., 2004; Semenza et al., 1997) and, more specifically, that verb constituents are more vulnerable to impairment than noun constituents in the production of compounds (e.g., Semenza et al., 1997), we also addressed the issue of the role of grammatical category in the performances of our participants. A comparison of adjectives and nouns in first- and second-constituent position across tasks did not yield differential results, indicating that, at least as far as compound processing is concerned, adjectives do not pose a higher degree of computational difficulty than nouns. Yet, in the aphasiological literature, adjectives have been found to be less stable than nouns in the production of complex adjectival noun phrases (e.g., Goodglass, 1993; Menn & Obler, 1990), pointing to the fact that mechanisms of word-internal syntax may differ from those of sentential syntax (for differential results on noun-adjective and adjective-noun sequences within compounds vs within noun phrases, see Mondini, Jarema, Luzzatti, Burani, & Semenza, 2002).

Our point of departure in this study was the assumption that compound production entails access to structural information at some level of lexical processing. Our findings demonstrating that position-in-the-string and compound headedness, as well as semantic specification of the more general constituent by the modifying constituent, influence error rates in the production of compounds by people with aphasia, supports this view from an as yet scarcely explored angle, that of bilingual performance. They are thus in line with previous neuropsychological studies showing compositional effects in compound production and strengthen the claim that morphological constituency does come into play during the processing of compound words. It is hoped that additional studies of compound processing in bilingual aphasia will further refine our understanding of the factors affecting the access of people with aphasia to these highly prevalent lexical constructs.

REFERENCES

Baayen, R. H., Piepenbrock, R., & Gulikers, L. (1995) *The CELEX lexical database* [CD-Rom]. Philadelphia: Linguistic Data Consortium, University of Pennsylvania.

Badecker, W. (2001). Lexical composition and the production of compounds: Evidence from errors in naming. *Language and Cognitive Processes, 16,* 337–366.

Blanken, G. (2000). The production of nominal compounds in aphasia. *Brain and Language, 74,* 84–102.

Content, A., Mousty, P., & Radeau, M. (1990). BRULEX: une base de données lexicales informatisées pour le français écrit et parlé. *L'Année Psychologique, 90,* 551–566.

Costa, A., Caramazza, A., & Sebastiàn-Gallés, N. (2000). The cognate facilitation effect: Implications for models of lexical access. *Journal of Experimental Psychology: Learning, Memory, and Cognition, 26,* 1283–1296.

de Bot, K., Cox, A., Ralston, S., Schaufeli, A., & Weltens, B. (1995). Lexical processing in bilinguals. *Second Language Research, 11,* 1–19.

de Groot, A. M. B., Borgwaldt, S., Bos, M., & van den Eijinden, E. (2002). Lexical decision and word naming in bilinguals: Language effects and task effects. *Journal of Memory and Language, 47,* 91–124.

Delazer, W., & Semenza, C. (1998). The processing of compound words: A study in aphasia. *Brain and Language, 61,* 54–62.

Dressler, W. U. (2006). Compound types. In G. Libben & G. Jarema (Eds.), *The representation and processing of compound words* (pp. 22–44). Oxford, UK: Oxford University Press.

Gagné, C. L. (2001). Relation and lexical priming during the interpretation of noun-noun combinations. *Journal of Experimental Psychology: Learning, Memory and Cognition, 27,* 236–254.

Gagné, C. L., & Shoben, E. J. (1997). The influence of thematic relation on the comprehension of modifier-noun combinations. *Journal of Experimental Psychology: Learning, Memory and Cognition, 23,* 71–87.

Gagné, C. L., & Spalding, T. L. (2006). Conceptual combination: Implication for the mental lexicon. In G. Libben & G. Jarema (Eds.), *The representation and processing of compound words* (pp. 145–168). Oxford, UK: Oxford University Press.

Goodglass, H. (1993). *Understanding aphasia.* San Diego, CA: Academic Press.

Hittmair-Delazer, M., Andrée, B., Semenza, C., de Bleser, R., & Benke, T. (1994). Naming by German compounds. *Journal of Neurolinguistics, 8,* 27–41.

Jarema, G., Busson, C., Nikolova, R., Tsapkini, K., & Libben, G. (1999). Processing compounds: A cross-linguistic study. *Brain and Language, 68,* 362–369.

Kaplan, K., & Goodglass, H. (1983). *The Boston Diagnostic Aphasia Examination.* Philadelphia: Lea & Febiger.

Kohnert, K. (2004). Cognitive and cognate-based treatments for bilingual aphasia: A case study. *Brain and Language, 91,* 294–302.

Lalor, E., & Kirsner, K. (2001). The representation of "false cognates" in the bilingual lexicon. *Psychonomic Bulletin and Review, 8,* 552–559.

Lecours, A. R., Nespoulous, J-L., Joanette, Y., Lemay, A., Puel, M., & Lafond, D. et al. (1986). *Protocole Montréal-Toulouse d'examen linguistique de l'aphasie. MT 86.* Montréal: Laboratoire Théophile-Alajouanine.

Libben, G., & Jarema, G. (Eds.). (2006). *The representation and processing of compound words.* Oxford, UK: Oxford University Press.

Mäkisalo, J., Niemi, J., & Laine, M. (1999). Finnish compound structure: Experiments with a morphologically impaired patient. *Brain and Language, 68,* 249–253.

Mazaux, J. M., & Orgogozo, J. M. (1982). *Échelle d'évaluation de l'aphasie (Boston Diagnostic Aphasia Examination) (BDAE).* Paris: Editions EAP.

Menn, L., & Obler, L. (Eds.). (1990). *Agrammatic aphasia: A cross-language narrative sourcebook.* Amsterdam: John Benjamins.

Mondini, S., Jarema, G., Luzzatti, C., Burani, C., & Semenza, C. (2002). Why is "Red Cross" different from "Yellow Cross"?: A neuropsychological study of noun-adjective agreement within Italian compounds. *Brain and Language, 81,* 621–634.

Mondini, S., Luzzatti, C., Zonca, G., Pistarini, C., & Semenza, C. (2004). The mental representation of verb-noun compounds in Italian: Evidence from a multiple single-case study in aphasia. *Brain and Language, 90,* 470–477.

Paradis, M. (1987). *The assessment of bilingual aphasia.* Hillsdale, NJ: Lawrence Erlbaum Associates Inc.

Roberts, P. M., & Deslauriers, L. (1999). Picture naming of cognate and non-cognate nouns in bilingual aphasia. *Journal of Communication Disorders, 32,* 1–22.

Schuell, H., & Sefer, J. W. (1973). *Differential diagnosis of aphasia with the Minnesota Test.* Minneapolis: University of Minnesota.

Semenza, C., Luzzatti, C., & Carabelli, S. (1997). Morphological representation of compound nouns: A study on Italian aphasic patients. *Journal of Neurolinguistics, 10,* 33–43.

Spencer, A. (1991). *Morphological theory.* Oxford, UK: Blackwell.

Stark, J., & Stark, H. K. (1990). On the processing of compounds nouns by Wernicke's aphasic. *Grazer Linguistische Studien, 35,* 95–113.

APPENDIX 1

EXAMPLES OF ERRORS

	French		English	
	Response	*Target*	*Response*	*Target*
Phonemic paraphasias	/kɛs blø/	(/kask blø/)	/næʃənl pɑːt/	(/næʃənl pɑːk/)
Morphological paraphasias	*lampe halogénique*	(lampe halogène)	*magical wand*	(magic wand)
Semantic paraphasias	*pois vert*	(haricot vert)	walk bridge	(promenade deck)
Verbal paraphasias	*occasion perdue*	(cause perdu)	*dead paper*	(dead leaf)
Neologisms	/tikɛ milt/	(/tikɛ R(ə)pɑ/)	/bas tʃɒklɪt/	(/hɒt tʃɒklɪt/)
Deletions of 1st or 2nd constituent	*carte –*	(carte-réponse)	- *shock*	(nervous shock)
Constituent inversion	basse marée	(marée basse)	*art dramatic*	(dramatic art)
Insertion of a preposition and/or a determiner	*assurance de vie*	(assurance-vie)	–	

APPENDIX 2

NUMBER OF ERRORS PER ERROR TYPE ON EACH TASK IN EACH LANGUAGE FOR PARTICIPANT RS

	French				English			
	Reading	*Repetition*	*Translation*	**Total**	*Reading*	*Repetition*	*Translation*	**Total**
Phonological	27	8	8	*44*	3	1	14	*18*
Morphological	17	1	11	*29*	2	0	3	*5*
Semantic	1	0	5	*6*	0	0	8	*8*
Missing	0	0	28	*28*	0	0	8	*8*
Neologism	1	0	0	*1*	0	0	0	*0*
Verbal	0	0	7	*7*	1	0	3	*4*
French*	0	0	0	*0*	0	0	9	*9*
English**	1	0	20	*21*	0	0	0	*0*
+Prep/+Det.	3	0	2	*5*	0	0	0	*0*
Inversion	0	0	6	*6*	0	0	19	*19*
Total	*50*	*9*	*87*	**146**	*6*	*1*	*64*	**71**

*French pronunciation of English word.   **English pronunciation of French word.

APPENDIX 3

NUMBER OF ERRORS PER ERROR TYPE ON EACH TASK IN EACH LANGUAGE FOR PARTICIPANT GK

	French				English			
	Reading	Repetition	Translation	Total	Reading	Repetition	Translation	Total
Phonological	6	6	5	17	1	0	0	1
Morphological	7	8	11	26	2	0	2	4
Semantic	0	0	11	11	0	0	12	12
Missing	0	0	31	31	0	2	7	9
Neologism	1	0	0	1	0	0	0	0
Verbal	0	0	5	5	0	0	0	0
French*	0	0	0	0	0	0	9	9
English**	0	0	1	1	0	0	0	0
+Prep/+Det.	2	0	6	8	0	0	0	0
Inversion	0	0	1	1	0	1	4	5
Total	16	14	71	101	3	3	34	40

*French pronunciation of English word.   **English pronunciation of French word.

APPENDIX 4

NUMBER OF ERRORS PER ERROR TYPE ON EACH TASK IN EACH LANGUAGE FOR PARTICIPANT VR

	French				English			
	Reading	Repetition	Translation	Total	Reading	Repetition	Translation	Total
Phonological	18	2	3	23	21	2	0	23
Morphological	1	0	0	1	0	1	1	2
Semantic	1	0	7	8	3	0	3	6
Missing	0	0	21	21	0	0	50	50
Neologism	0	0	1	1	0	0	0	0
Verbal	0	0	2	2	0	0	1	1
French*	0	0	1	1	2	0	2	4
English**	0	0	0	0	0	0	0	0
+Prep/+Det.	0	0	0	0	0	0	0	0
Inversion	0	0	3	3	0	0	1	1
Total	20	2	38	60	26	3	58	87

*French pronunciation of English word.   **English pronunciation of French word.

APHASIOLOGY, 2010, 24 (2), 141–169

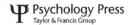

Psychology Press
Taylor & Francis Group

On the translation routes in early and highly proficient bilingual people: Evidence from an individual with semantic impairment

Mireia Hernández,[1] Albert Costa,[2] Agnès Caño,[1]
Montserrat Juncadella,[3] and Jordi Gascón-Bayarri[3]

[1]*Departament de Psicologia Bàsica, Universitat de Barcelona, Spain,* [2]*ICREA &
Departament de Tecnologies de la Informació i les Comunicacions, Universitat Pompea
Fabra, Barcelona, Spain, and* [3]*Unitat de Diagnòstic i Tractament de Demències,
Servei de Neurologia de l'Hospital Universitari de Bellvitge, Spain*

Background: One of the major interests in bilingualism research has been the extent to which the two lexicons of a bilingual speaker are directly linked and the role that this hypothetical link plays during language production. Up to now, most of the research on this issue has focused on either low or high proficient late-bilingual people, whereas little information has been provided on the functionality of this hypothesised link in highly proficient bilinguals who acquired their two languages early in life.
Aims: The aim of the present study is to provide information on the functionality of the direct link between the two lexicons of early and highly proficient bilingual people.
Methods & Procedures: In this report we assess the functionality of lexical links between translation words in an early and highly proficient Catalan–Spanish bilingual patient (JFF) who suffers from a semantic deficit as a consequence of Alzheimer's disease. The integrity of JFF's conceptual and lexical representations is examined by means of semantic, picture-naming, and translation tasks. We pay special attention to JFF's translation performance to assess whether such performance is affected by his semantic deficit.
Outcomes & Results: We argue that if lexical links between translation words are functional, then such links would guarantee error-free production in translation. Contrary to this prediction, errors observed in JFF's translation performance indicated that the semantic system was involved in JFF's forward and backward translation.
Conclusions: On the basis of this result, we suggest that lexical links in early and highly proficient bilingual people are not functional.

Keywords: Bilingualism; Lexical routes; Semantic impairment.

Address correspondence to: Albert Costa, Department de Tecnologies de la Informació i les Comunicacions, Universitat Pompeu Fabra, C. Roc Boronat 138, Barcelona, Spain. E-mail: costalbert@ gmail.com

The authors are grateful to Ms Ivanova for her comments on previous versions of this manuscript. This research was supported by two grants from the Spanish Government (SEJ -2005/CONSOLIDER-INGENIO). Mireia Hernández was supported by a pre-doctoral fellowship from the Catalan Government.

http://www.psypress.com/aphasiology   DOI: 10.1080/02687030902958266

The functional architecture of the two lexicons of bilingual speakers has been an issue of intense research in the last 30 years (e.g., Beauvillain & Grainger, 1987; Chen, 1992; Chen & Leung, 1989; Cheung & Chen, 1998; Cristoffanini, Kirsner, & Milech, 1986; de Groot, Dannenburg, & van Hell, 1994; Grainger & Beauvillain, 1988; Kirsner, Smith, Lockart, King, & Jain, 1984; Hernández, Caño, Costa, Sebastián-Gallés, Juncadella, & Gascón-Bayarri, 2008; Hernández, Costa, Sebastián-Gallés, Juncadella, & Reñé, 2007; Kroll & Stewart, 1994; La Heij et al., 1990; La Heij, Hooglander, Kerling & van der Velden, 1996; Poncelet, Majerus, Raman, Warginaire, & Weekes, 2007; Potter, So, von Eckart, & Feldman, 1984; Sanchez-Casas, Davis, & Garcia-Albea, 1992; Sholl, Sankaranarayanan, & Kroll, 1995; Van Hell & De Groot, 1998; Van Hell & Dijkstra, 2002; see also the recent handbook on bilingualism by Kroll & De Groot, 2005).

A particular question that has been hotly debated is the extent to which lexical representations of the bilingual person's two languages are connected with each other at the lexical level. That is, the issue is whether translation equivalents are in some way directly linked to each other at the lexical level (see Figure 1), and if so, what function such a link has during language processing. Most of the research assessing the functionality of lexical links has explored the performance of either low or highly proficient *late* bilingual people (that is, those who did not acquire their L2 until at least late childhood or early adulthood, achieving either a low or high level of proficiency)—little work has been done to assess the presence of such links for bilingual people who acquired two languages early in life and then attain high proficiency in L2. The main goal of this article is to provide new clues concerning the functionality of direct lexical links between translation equivalents in early and highly proficient bilinguals. To do so we assess the translation performance of an early and highly proficient bilingual speaker (JFF) suffering from Alzheimer's disease (AD).

First, we provide an overview of the theoretical views on the existence of lexical links and the experimental evidence (mostly coming from late bilingual people) that has been used to support such views. Second, we put forward the hypothesis that lexical links may also become functional in the case of early and highly proficient bilingual people. Third, we test this hypothesis by analysing the linguistic performance of an early and highly proficient bilingual patient with a semantic impairment due to AD.

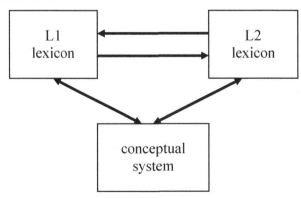

Figure 1. Schematic representation of the translation routes. Translation may be achieved through direct links between the two lexicons (the word association hypothesis) or via the shared conceptual system (the concept mediation hypothesis).

LEXICAL LINKS BETWEEN TRANSLATION WORDS IN LATE BILINGUAL PEOPLE

Models of bilingual language processing have postulated the existence of links between translation words and have also made explicit claims about the role of two variables on their functionality. First, L2 lexical representations tend to be more strongly connected to L1 lexical representations than vice versa (e.g., Kroll & Stewart, 1994; La Heij et al., 1996). This claim is based on the notion that during the first stages of L2 learning, access to the meaning of L2 words is mediated by previous access to the L1 lexical representations (Chen & Leung, 1989; Kroll & Curley, 1988). In contrast, access to the semantic system for L1 words is not mediated by prior access to L2 representations. Consequently, the links between L2 and L1 should be more functional than those between L1 and L2. Second, this asymmetry in the functionality of the lexical links appears to apply primarily to those bilingual speakers who acquire their L2 under formal instruction and relatively late.

The experimental evidence regarding the functionality of lexical links has come primarily from translation studies and, specifically, whether word translation can (or cannot) bypass the semantic system. Given the framework presented in Figure 1, in principle, word translation can be achieved through two different routes. First, a word in one language (the prompt word) can be translated into its corresponding version (the response word) by retrieving its meaning and using such information to access the corresponding word in the other (the response) language. This route is often referred to as the "concept mediation route" (or hypothesis). Second, word translation can also be achieved by a direct link between translation words. That is, the prompt word, once it is presented, would automatically send activation to its corresponding translation in the response language. In such a situation, the speaker only needs to select the word in the response language that is most activated, which usually corresponds (in error-free translation) to the correct translation word. This route is usually referred to as the "word association route" (or hypothesis). Note that, in the strong version of this latter hypothesis, whether or not the prompt word has access to its semantic representation is irrelevant for the translation process. That is, in principle, a speaker with a semantic deficit might be able to perform a translation task without problems, by means of the lexical links between translation words. It is important to note that these two routes are not mutually exclusive and that both of them might be concurrently functional in the process of word translation. That is, both the word association route and the concept mediation route may be engaged in word translation, reinforcing each other, at least in error-free translation performance. As we will see, the possibility that both routes are functional is a fundamental issue to be considered, especially when assessing the translation performance of early and highly proficient bilingual speakers.

Most of the evidence put forward regarding two routes for translation comes from the presence/absence of semantic effects in translation tasks (e.g., de Groot, 1992; de Groot et al., 1994; Duyck & Brysbaert, 2008; Kroll & Stewart, 1994; La Heij et al., 1990, 1996; Sholl et al., 1995). The logic of these studies is the following. If performance in a translation task is affected by semantic factors, then this is taken as evidence that the semantic system has played a role in the translation process. Alternatively, if such translation performance is not affected by semantic factors, then this is taken as evidence that translation has been performed through the lexical links between lexical representations, hence bypassing the semantic system.

Given the assumed asymmetry between the strength of the lexical links from L1 to L2 and vice versa, the existence of semantic effects affecting the translation process needs to be assessed in relation to the direction of the translation process. Forward translation refers to the process by which a word is translated from the dominant language into the non-dominant language, while backward translation refers to the opposite translation direction. As described above, the claims made about the functionality of lexical links depend on the direction of the translation process, such functionality being greater in backward than in forward translation.

There seems to be a consensus regarding the involvement of the semantic system in forward translation. In a seminal study Kroll and Stewart (1994) asked participants to translate two types of word lists. In the "semantically blocked" lists all words belonged to the same semantic category, while in the "semantically heterogeneous" lists the words belonged to different semantic categories. Importantly, in forward translation, response latencies were slower in the homogeneous lists than in the heterogeneous lists, revealing a semantic interference effect (see Brown, 1981; Damian, Vigliocco & Levelt, 2001; Kroll & Curley, 1988). Given this semantic interference effect, Kroll and Stewart concluded that forward translation is mainly conceptually mediated. A similar conclusion was reached by La Heij et al. (1996) in a series of Stroop-like translation experiments. In these experiments participants were presented with a prompt word and a distractor picture that had to be ignored—i.e., the word to be translated (e.g., shark) was presented along with a picture that might be semantically related (e.g., whale) or unrelated (e.g., carrot) with that word. The results of these experiments showed that when the prompt word was semantically related to the distractor picture, translation times were faster than when the prompt word was unrelated, suggesting that word translation had been achieved through the semantic system (see also Altarriba & Mathis, 1997, Bloem & La Heij, 2003).

More controversial is the issue of whether translation from L2 into L1 (backward translation) is actually performed through word association, therefore bypassing the semantic system. Indeed, whether or not this is the case is fundamental for postulating the existence of lexical links between translation words. The debate regarding this issue revolves on whether the presence of semantic effects in backward translation is a reliable phenomenon. Although some authors have shown semantic effects in similar paradigms as the ones described above (e.g., de Groot & Poot, 1997; de Groot et al., 1994; La Heij et al., 1990, 1996), others have failed to do so (Kroll & Stewart, 1994; Sholl et al., 1995). Thus, and despite several differences in the paradigms used in these studies, the question still remains of whether (or under which conditions) backward translation can be performed through direct links between translation words, bypassing the semantic system.

LEXICAL LINKS BETWEEN TRANSLATION WORDS IN EARLY AND HIGHLY PROFICIENT BILINGUAL PEOPLE

As described above, the claim that functional lexical links exist between translation words has been put forward most strongly for cases in which the L2 is acquired relatively late in life and through formal instruction. Also, L2 proficiency is a factor that is assumed to affect the functionality of such links. Accordingly, for those proficient bilingual speakers who have acquired their L2 early in life, the role of lexical links might be minimal. This is because, for these bilingual speakers, access to the semantic system from L2 representations does not need involve prior access to L1 representations given that the two languages have been acquired almost simultaneously.

However, it is possible that lexical links between translation words are also the result of other computational processes than those engaged in formal instruction. In the case of early and highly proficient bilingual speakers who use their two languages on an everyday basis, such a computational process may be the co-activation of their two languages during language processing. Let us elaborate this point a bit further. There is ample evidence suggesting the co-activation of the two languages of a bilingual person during language production and perception (e.g., Costa & Caramazza, 1999; Costa, La Heij, & Navarrete, 2006a; Costa, Miozzo, & Caramazza, 1999; de Bot & Schreuder, 1992; Dijkstra & Van Heuven, 2002; Duyck, Assche, Drieghe, & Hartsuiker, 2007; Green, 1986, 1998; Hermans, Bongaerts, de Bot, & Schreuder, 1998; La Heij, 2005; Poulisse & Bongaerts, 1994; Rodriguez-Fornells, van der Lugt, & Rotte, 2005). For example, every time a word is produced in language A, the translation word in Language B is also activated to some extent. In fact, in the case of speech production, there is some evidence that the phonological activation of the intended word in Language A re-activates not only lexical representations belonging to Language A but also those belonging to Language B (Costa, Roelstraete, & Hartsuiker, 2006b). Thus there seems to be a reverberation between the two lexicons such that, when there is the intention of producing a word in Language A, this leads to the automatic activation of its translation in Language B. This could, in principle, lead to the development of functional lexical links between translation words. It is important to note here that such a reverberation will be maximal for highly proficient bilingual speakers, given that the parallel activation of the two languages is present regardless of the language they use for communication, while for low-proficient bilingual speakers activation of the weak language may be minimal when speaking in the dominant language. Consequently, one may think that it is precisely in early and highly proficient bilingual people where direct connections between translation words would be maximally functional. The objective of our study is to assess the functionality of lexical links in early and highly proficient bilingual people.

Given the discussion about the asymmetries in the presence of lexical links between the two lexicons, it is important to mention here that, in principle, these asymmetries should not be present in the case of early and highly proficient bilingual speakers. This is because the computational process that leads to the presence of such links for these bilingual people works similarly when using either of the two languages. That is, there is always co-activation of the two languages of a bilingual person regardless of the language being used. Thus, for these bilingual people, the lexical links between the two languages should be of the same strength.

The number of studies addressing the functionality of lexical links in early and highly proficient bilingual speakers is relatively small, and has led to relatively inconsistent results. Most of these studies have used cross-linguistic semantic and translation priming, but little consistency exists across them (see Kiran & Lebel, 2007, for a summary of the cross-linguistic semantic and translation priming studies from 1974 to 2007). The inconsistency is apparent in whether semantic priming is present or not in backward translation, and it has been argued that methodological differences may be behind such inconsistency (see Basnight-Brown & Altarriba, 2007, for a review on these methodological concerns). In a recent study,

Basnight-Brown and Altarriba (2007) explored the performance of early and highly proficient Spanish–English bilingual speakers with a more dominant L2 (English) in semantic and translation priming experiments. These authors found significant translation priming for both language directions but significant semantic priming only from L2 (English) to L1 (Spanish). Kiran and Lebel (2007) also administered semantic priming and translation priming tasks to early highly proficient Spanish–English bilingual speakers who have shifted their language dominance from L1 to L2. These participants were classified into two groups according to the grade of language dominance (more-balanced and less-balanced bilingual speakers). The most relevant observation of this study was that the more-balanced group showed translation priming effects only from L2 (English) to L1 (Spanish), whereas the less-balanced group obtained translation priming effects in both translation directions. In line with Heredia (1995, 1996), these observations suggest that priming effects arise from the more-dominant to the less-dominant language, regardless of which of them has been acquired first.

Although these results are interesting, they are silent regarding the issue tackled in our study. This is because the participants tested in these studies typically reside in English-dominant language environments and therefore have usually shifted their language dominance from L1 (Spanish) to L2 (English). One purpose of our study is to examine the functionality of the lexical links in an early and highly proficient Catalan (L1) – Spanish (L2) bilingual person without language dominance shift residing in a balanced language environment.

An important problem when assessing the functionality of the lexical links is that both the lexical and the conceptual route may be engaged concurrently during the translation task. This is a problem when assessing the performance of any bilingual speaker, but it is certainly more important in the case of early and highly proficient bilingual people, given that for these speakers lexical representations of both languages are presumably robustly connected to the semantic system. If this is so, it would be very difficult to find any experimental situation in which normal speakers do not reveal a semantic effect in translation tasks. However, this observation does not mean that lexical links are not functional per se; it only shows that the conceptual route is functional. Perhaps a more promising way to assess whether the lexical links are functional is to find a situation in which the translation product of the concept mediation route conflicts with the translation product of the lexical route. For example, if the concept mediation route leads to the retrieval of a wrong translation word and the lexical route leads to the retrieval of the correct translation word, then it would be possible to assess whether the bilingual person ends up blocking the incorrect production. The objective of the present report is to test this exact issue.

To address this issue we report the performance of an early and highly proficient bilingual speaker (JFF) who shows a semantic deficit due to AD. There are two straightforward predictions that one can put forward regarding the performance of JFF in word translation. First, if word translation engages the conceptual route then we should expect semantic errors in word translation. Second, if word translation engages the word association route then we should expect correct responses, provided that the lexical links are not damaged.

These two hypotheses need to be taken cautiously, however, because of the potential contribution of both routes to the translation task. That is, it is possible that translation engages the two routes presented above, namely the word association and the concept mediation route. As discussed above, in normal speakers both routes will be functional and hence translation may be achieved by any of them, reducing therefore the presence (or detectability) of semantic effects. In the case of a patient with damage to the semantic system, given that the connections between translation words should be functional for this speaker, the result of the translation via the conceptual route and via the word association route will lead to two different responses—a semantically related (wrong) word and the correct word. In such a scenario one may expect either the production of the correct word or a non-response. This is because the semantic error generated from the concept mediation route will be blocked by the activation of the correct translation word via the word association route (see Figure 2) (similar arguments are made to explain semantic errors in deep dyslexia).

To sum up, positive evidence for the presence of lexical links between translation words will be gathered if JFF is able to perform the translation task without errors or, less convincingly, if non-responses are produced rather than semantic errors (showing the blocking of the semantic error). Following this logic, if we find that JFF commits semantic errors in translation, then we could argue that the concept mediation route is functional (generating the semantic error) and the word association route is not functional (does not prevent the production of the semantic error).

CASE REPORT

JFF was an 81-year-old right-handed Catalan–Spanish bilingual speaker who worked as a carpenter from the time he finished primary school until his retirement. His L1 was Catalan, but he was exposed to Spanish (L2) at a very early age; his schooling was in Spanish and he used this language on a daily basis throughout his life (see Appendix A for a detailed description of JFF's language use). JFF had been diagnosed with AD 7 years before testing for the present study. The most important neuropsychological findings were personal and temporo-spatial disorientation and episodic memory impairment. JFF's spontaneous language was fluent without grammatical errors or paraphasias. Neither he nor any member of his family reported anomia or any problem in recognising objects. Tests for the present study were conducted in the course of 2005 (see Appendix B for a description of JFF's neuropsychological profile).

Exploring JFF's conceptual system

JFF's conceptual knowledge was assessed through the Pyramids and Palm Trees Test (Howard & Patterson, 1992), as well as through an adaptation into Spanish of the verbal questionnaire developed by Laiacona, Barbarotto, Trivelli, and Capitani (1993). JFF's performance on both tasks evidenced a clear impairment of the conceptual system.

Pyramids and Palm Trees Test. In this task JFF had to decide which of the two pictures presented as response options was conceptually associated to a third picture (target stimulus). The two response options were semantically related, but only one of them was associated to the target picture. JFF had to point to the response picture that was associated to the target. JFF was able to give only 73% correct responses

Case 1

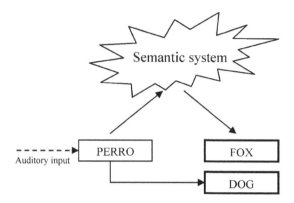

Case 2

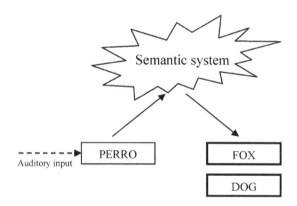

Figure 2. Schematic representation of translation performances of a hypothetical early and highly proficient Spanish–English bilingual person with damage to the semantic system. Case 1: If direct lexical links between the two lexicons were functional, then those links should block the production of semantic errors in translation (e.g., the word "perro" would be correctly translated into "dog", bypassing the impaired semantic system). Case 2: If direct lexical links between the two lexicons were not functional, then semantic errors would be detected in translation (e.g. the word "perro" would be translated into "fox" instead of "dog").

(38/52 trials), thus putting him below the normal range for his age and education level (94% correct) according to Spanish normative data (Rami et al., 2008).

Semantic memory questionnaire. In this task JFF was asked six questions about each of the 60 items included in this questionnaire. Questions required a forced-choice response with three alternatives that were semantically related (e.g., Does a cow give milk, eggs, or wool?). Each correct response counted as 1 point, leading to a maximum score of 360 points. JFF's performance was compared to that of two healthy control participants matched in age and years of education to JFF (AS: 79 years old, 9 years of education; AU: 77 years old, 6 years of education). JFF's performance was significantly worse than that of the other two control participants (JFF: 262/360, 73% correct/AS: 346/360, 96% correct; $\chi^2 = 75.84$, $p = .0001$/AU: 351/360, 98% correct; $\chi^2 = 88.24$, $p = .0001$). As an example, JFF responded "flies" to the question of whether a mouse runs, flies, or swims.

In sum, JFF's performance in the two tasks that explored the semantic system (Pyramids and Palm Trees Test and the semantic memory questionnaire) was lower than normal, suggesting the presence of a semantic deficit associated with dementia. In the following we explore to what extent this impairment affected picture-naming and translation tasks.

JFF's picture-naming performance in L1 and L2

JFF was presented with a set of 62 black-and-white line drawings (see Appendix C for a detailed description of these materials). JFF was asked to name the pictures in two different sessions 2 days apart. He performed the task in L1 (Catalan) in the first session and in L2 (Spanish) in the second.

JFF's naming performance was similarly impaired in the two languages (L1: 42% correct, L2: 31% correct; $\chi^2 = 1.71$, $p = .19$).

Of special interest is the type of errors committed by JFF in the naming task. The errors were classified into two main types: semantic (SEM) and inappropriate word forms (IWF) (see Appendix D for the transcription and classification of all JFF's errors). An error was classified as semantic if JFF produced a word that was semantically related to the target, or when he started producing several words that were semantically related to the target, or when he gave some semantic information (category membership or some property) about the target but was unable to come up with the response. These errors may stem from his semantic deficit or from a failure to retrieve the correct lexical representation.

Errors were classified as IWF when JFF produced the word in the non-target language. There were also some "don't know" responses, which were classified as non-responses (NR). No other types of errors were registered.

As expected, most of the errors in L1 and L2 picture naming were semantic errors (L1: 27/36, 75% of errors, L2: 30/43, 70% of errors), while only very few errors consisted of IWF (L1: 0/36, 0% of errors; L2: 3/43, 7% of errors) or non-responses (L1: 9/36, 25% of errors; L2: 10/43, 23% of errors) (see Figure 3). Interestingly, JFF's performance in this task was not affected by the cognate status of the picture names either in L1 (cognates: 35% correct, non-cognates: 48% correct; $\chi^2 = 1.06$, $p = .3$) or in L2 (cognates: 23% correct, non-cognates: 39% correct; $\chi^2 = 1.9$, $p = .17$). The lack of a cognate effect in a patient with a semantic deficit is consistent with the hypothesis of a phonological origin of cognate effects (see Costa, Santesteban, & Caño, 2005).

In sum, JFF's naming problems are present in both languages, a result that is consistent with a semantic origin of these naming problems. A critical question is whether this semantic impairment can be detected in translation.

JFF's performance on forward and backward translation

JFF was asked to translate the same set of 62 items used in the picture-naming tasks in two different sessions 2 days apart. The prompt words were spoken by the experimenter and JFF gave his response orally. This testing started a week after the

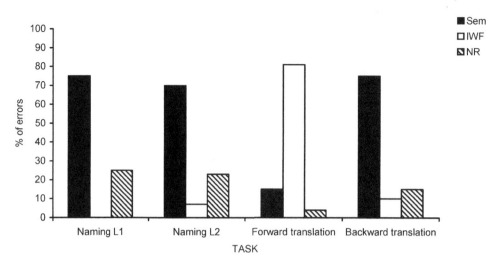

Figure 3. Proportion of each type of error JFF made in the picture naming and translation tasks.

end of the picture-naming sessions. In the first session JFF performed a forward translation task; that is, from L1 (Catalan) to L2 (Spanish). In the second session, JFF was asked to perform a backward translation task; that is, from L2 (Spanish) to L1 (Catalan). The target words were read aloud by the experimenter, who was also a highly proficient bilingual speaker.

JFF's performance in forward and backward translation was clearly impaired. He was able to translate only 56% of the items in forward and only 68% in backward translation, the amount of impairment being similar in both tasks ($\chi^2 = 1.68$, $p = .19$). As expected, JFF was more accurate translating cognate than non-cognate words, both translating into L1 (cognates: 84% correct, non-cognates: 52% correct, $\chi^2 = 7.38$, $p = .007$) and into L2 (cognates: 77%, non-cognates: 35%, $\chi^2 = 11.1$, $p = .001$) (see de Groot, 1992; Sánchez-Casas et al., 1992; for a revision of the cognate effect in translation). This is the reason why the level of performance in translation was greater than in picture naming. This cognate effect in translation contrasts with its absence in the picture-naming task.

Of special relevance for the present study is the pattern of errors committed by JFF in the translation task (see Appendix D for the transcription and classification of all of JFF's errors). Errors were classified following the same criteria used in the picture-naming task. However, in the IWF we also included instances in which JFF tried to translate the target word by adding or removing some phonological material, leading to a nonword. For example, he translated "mussol" into "mussuelo" (see below).

The main pattern of errors in forward translation consisted of producing IWF (*SEM*: 4/27, 15% of errors; IWF: 22/27, 81% of errors; NR: 1/27, 4% of errors) (see Figure 3). Most of the IWF corresponded with regularisations of the L1 non-cognate word as if it were a cognate—e.g., instead of translating "mussol" (L1 word for *owl*) into "*búho*" (L2 word for *owl*), he translated "mussol" into "mussuelo (stem of L1 word inflection)". That is, JFF seems to adopt the strategy of adapting the target word to the response language by adding some suffixes. However this strategy results in nonwords, revealing that JFF is simply guessing the response word. There were also some errors in which JFF's response in L2 was identical to the L1 presented word.

A crucial observation for our study is that the errors in the backward translation task were mostly semantic (*SEM*: 15/20, 75% of errors; IWF: 2/20, 10% of errors; NR: 3/20, 15% of errors) (see Figure 3). This observation in backward translation demonstrates that this translation process was semantically mediated, and that the lexical links between L2 and L1 were not functional enough to block the retrieval of the incorrect translation.

GENERAL DISCUSSION

In this paper our aim was to explore the functionality of the hypothesised lexical links between translation words in early and highly proficient bilingual speakers. As described in the introduction, some models of bilingual lexical access assume the existence of direct links between the lexical representations of the relatively proficient late bilingual speaker's two languages.

To assess whether such links are functionally developed in early and highly proficient bilingual people we tested the performance of an early and highly proficient bilingual speaker who suffered from AD. JFF showed poor performance in several tasks that required access to the semantic system (picture naming, Pyramids and Palm Trees Test), suggesting the presence of damage to this system as a consequence of the disease.

More important for our purposes is the low performance (about 60% correct) exhibited by JFF in the translation task, and particularly the pattern of errors (mostly semantic errors and phonological adaptations of the to-be-translated word). These results contrast with the predictions derived from the hypothesis of the functionality of lexical links between translation words. Recall that if lexical links are functional then one should expect either the production of the correct translation words, or possibly non-responses due to the elicitation of two answers (one coming from the semantic system and a different one coming from the word association route). Hence we do not find positive evidence about the involvement of the word association route in the performance of JFF.

There is, however, a somewhat unexpected result in the pattern of errors observed in forward and backward translation. In backward translation (from L2 to L1) most of the errors were semantic substitutions, suggesting the influence of damage to the semantic system in this task. However, the errors in forward translation (from L1 to L2) were mostly phonological adaptations of the to-be-translated word. That is, JFF gave as answers adaptations of the L1 prompt word that resulted in non-existing words in both the prompt and the response language. What is the origin of such differential behaviour in the two directions of translation? If the translation process involves the concept mediation route, then one should expect JFF to produce semantic errors in both directions of translation. Before presenting a tentative explanation for this performance, it is important to stress that the phonological adaptations of the to-be-translated word are unlikely to stem from the existence of lexical links between translation words. This is because the functioning of lexical links should have led to the production of the correct lexical representation. This is far from what JFF does. Rather, he does not seem to have access to the translation word at all, and then he generates a phonological adaptation of the prompt word to accommodate it (more or less) to the Spanish phonology.

A tentative explanation of the origin of these errors is that damage to the semantic system has a larger effect in access to L2 lexical representations than to L1 lexical representations. That is, given semantic damage, access to the lexicon from the semantic system may affect the two languages to a different extent. In other words, when retrieving a word in L1, a semantic deficit may lead to an abnormal activation of the lexical system that results in the selection of a semantically related word. However, if we assume that lexical access in L2 is less robust than in L1, then it is possible that the abnormal activation of the lexical system results in not enough activation of any lexical form and consequently lexical selection cannot proceed. In these instances, JFF may be unable to select any word (the correct one or a semantically related one) in L2. However, given the similarities between the lexical representations of JFF's two languages (Spanish and Catalan), with a large number of cognate words, JFF may have developed the strategy of trying to adapt the phonological content of the prompt word to the Spanish phonology in order to give a response. In some cases this strategy may lead to the correct response, provided that JFF's metalinguistic knowledge of how to apply the phonological adaptations is precise enough. However, in many other cases these adaptations lead to the production of non-responses.

Although this is a tentative explanation, what is important for our purposes is that the performance of JFF in forward and backward translation does not reveal any trace of the involvement of lexical links between translation words.

A potential caveat when interpreting our findings refers to whether JFF's performance reveals damage to the lexical links between translation words or rather reveals the absence of such links to begin with. That is, it is possible that early and highly proficient bilingual speakers do not develop lexical links between translation words during language learning (or processing), and consequently they always achieve translation through the semantic system. This is indeed what appears to be the consensus in the psycholinguistic literature (e.g., Duyck & Brysbaert, 2007), in the sense that the links between lexical representations would be a consequence of a late and formal learning of the L2 words. Thus, whether or not such links also exist in early and highly proficient unimpaired bilingual speakers is still an open question.

However, such a question would be very hard to answer by testing unimpaired bilingual speakers. This is because, as discussed in the introduction, it is possible that both routes of translation are functional in these bilingual people. If so, it will be very difficult not to detect semantic effects during translation. A more promising avenue to answer this question is to test bilingual people who have deficits to the semantic system and assess whether the lexical links can block the semantic errors resulting from the semantic damage.[1] This is precisely the contribution of our study. In fact, if functional links are actually established for this type of bilingual speaker, then one should be able to find patients who make use of such links to prevent the production of semantic errors. This is because the effects of brain damage may not impair the cognitive system in a complete manner, but rather in a more progressive way, allowing the detection of the functionality of a lexical route in translation.

---

[1] Although the specific origin of the semantic impairment of an individual may lead to different patterns of semantic deterioration, the logic of our study would apply to any patient with semantic deficits that lead to semantic errors in language production. Consequently, we predict that the observed pattern of results would be also present in other patients with semantic deficits that are not due to AD.

Before concluding, it is important to stress that the similarities between the two languages of a bilingual person might play a role in the likelihood of developing lexical links between translation words. One possibility is that the more similar the formal properties between the translation words of the two languages, the more likely the instantiation of lexical links. On this view, languages with a large number of cognate words would provide the best test for the presence of lexical links. This is precisely the case in Catalan and Spanish, for which about 70% of the translation words are cognates. Consequently, given the results observed in our study, we might predict the involvement of the semantic system in the translation processes in early and highly proficient bilingual speakers of more dissimilar languages.

To conclude, the present research suggests that the functional architecture of early and highly proficient bilingual speakers is one in which the lexical links between translation words do not seem to play any functional role. However, in our view, data provided in the present article need to be taken as a starting point for future research on the issue.

REFERENCES

Altarriba, J., & Mathis, K. M. (1997). Conceptual and lexical development in second language acquisition. *Journal of Memory & Language, 36*, 550–568.

Basnight-Brown, D. M., & Altarriba, J. (2007). Differences in semantic and translation priming across languages: The role of language direction and language dominance. *Memory & Cognition, 35*(5), 953–965.

Beauvillain, C., & Grainger, J. (1987). Accessing interlexical homographs: Some limitations of a language-selective access. *Journal of Memory and Language, 26*, 658–672.

Bloem, I., & La Heij, W. (2003). Semantic facilitation and semantic interference in word translation: Implications for models of lexical access in language production. *Journal of Memory and Language, 48*, 468–488.

Brown, A. S. (1981). Inhibition in cued retrieval. *Journal of Experimental Psychology: Human Learning and Memory, 7*, 204–215.

Chen, H. C. (1992). Lexical processing in bilingual or multilingual speakers. In R. J. Harris (Ed.), *Cognitive processing in bilinguals* (pp. 253–264). Amsterdam: North Holland.

Chen, H. C., & Leung, Y. S. (1989). Patterns of lexical processing in a non-native language. *Journal of Experimental Psychology: Learning, Memory, & Cognition, 15*, 316–325.

Cheung, H., & Chen, H. C. (1998). Lexical and conceptual processing in Chinese–English bilinguals: Further evidence for asymmetry. *Memory & Cognition, 26*, 1002–1013.

Costa, A., & Caramazza, A. (1999). Is lexical selection in bilingual speech production language specific? Further evidence from Spanish–English and English–Spanish bilinguals. *Bilingualism: Language and Cognition, 2*(3), 231–244.

Costa, A., La Heij, W., & Navarrete, E. (2006a). The dynamics of bilingual lexical access. *Bilingualism: Language and Cognition, 9*(2), 137–151.

Costa, A., Miozzo, M., & Caramazza, A. (1999). Lexical selection in bilinguals: Do words in the bilingual's two lexicons compete for selection? *Journal of Memory and Language, 41*, 365–397.

Costa, A., Roelstraete, B., & Hartsuiker, R. (2006b). The lexical bias effect in bilingual speech production: Evidence for feedback between lexical and sublexical levels across languages. *Psychonomic Bulletin & Review, 13*, 612–617.

Costa, A., Santesteban, M., & Caño, A. (2005). On the facilitatory effects of cognate words in bilingual speech production. *Brain and Language, 94*, 94–103.

Cristoffanini, P., Kirsner, K., & Milech, D. (1986). Bilingual lexical representation: The status of Spanish–English cognates. *The Quarterly Journal of Experimental Psychology, 38A*, 367–393.

Damian, M. F., Vigliocco, G., & Levelt, W. J. M. (2001). Effects of semantic context in the naming of pictures and words. *Cognition, 81*(3), B77–87.

de Bot, K., & Schreuder, R. (1992). Word production and the bilingual lexicon. In R. Schreuder & B. Weltens (Eds.), *The bilingual lexicon* (pp. 191–214). Amsterdam, Netherlands: John Benjamins Publishing Company.

de Groot, A. M. (1992). Determinants of word translation. *Journal of Experimental Psychology: Learning, Memory, & Cognition, 18*, 1001–1018.

de Groot, A. M. B., Dannenburg, L., & van Hell, J. G. (1994). Forward and backward word translation by bilinguals. *Journal of Memory and Language, 33*, 600–629.

de Groot, A. M. B., & Poot, R. (1997). Word translation at three levels of proficiency in a second language: The ubiquitous involvement of conceptual memory. *Language Learning, 47*, 215–264.

Dijkstra, A. F. J., & Van Heuven, W. J. B. (2002). The architecture of the bilingual word recognition system: From identification to decision. *Bilingualism: Language and Cognition, 5*(3), 175–197.

Duyck, W., Assche, E., Drieghe, D., & Hartsuiker, R. J. (2007). Visual word recognition by bilinguals in a sentence context: Evidence for nonselective lexical access. *Journal of Experimental Psychology: Learning, Memory, and Cognition, 33*, 663–679.

Duyck, W., & Brysbaert, M. (2007). Forward and backward number translation requires conceptual mediation in both balanced and unbalanced bilinguals. *Journal of Experimental Psychology: Human Perception and Performance, 30*, 889–906.

Duyck, W., & Brysbaert, M. (2008). Semantic access in number word translation: The role of crosslingual lexical similarity. *Experimental Psychology, 55*, 102–112.

Folstein, M. F., Folstein, S. E., & McHugh, P. R. (1975). "Mini-mental state". A practical method for grading the cognitive state of patients for the clinician. *Journal of Psychiatric Research, 12*(3), 189–198.

Grainger, J., & Beauvillain, C. (1988). Associative priming in bilinguals: Some limits of interlingual facilitation effects. *Canadian Journal of Psychology, 42*(3), 261–273.

Green, D. W. (1986). Control, activation and resource. *Brain and Language, 27*, 210–223.

Green, D. W. (1998). Mental control of the bilingual lexico-semantic system. *Bilingualism: Language and Cognition, 1*, 67–81.

Heredia, R. R. (1995). *Concreteness effects in high frequency words: A test of the revised hierarchical and the mixed models of bilingual memory representations.* Unpublished Doctoral Dissertation, University of California, Santa Cruz.

Heredia, R. R. (1996, 10 January). Bilingual memory: A re-revised version of the hierarchical model of bilingual memory. In *The Newsletter of the Centre for Research in Language:* University of California, San Diego.

Hermans, D., Bongaerts, T., de Bot, K., & Schreuder, R. (1998). Producing words in a foreign language: Can speakers prevent interference from their first language? *Bilingualism, 1*, 213–229.

Hernández, M., Caño, A., Costa, A., Sebastián-Gallés, N., Juncadella, M., & Gascón-Bayarri, J. (2008). Grammatical category-specific deficits in bilingual aphasia. *Brain and Language*.

Hernández, M., Costa, A., Sebastián-Gallés, N., Juncadella, M., & Reñé, R. (2007). The organization of nouns and verbs in bilingual speakers: A case of bilingual grammatical category-specific deficit. *Journal of Neurolinguistics, 20*, 285–305.

Howard, D., & Patterson, K. (1992). *The Pyramids and Palm Trees Test.* Windsor, UK: Thames Valley Test Company.

Kiran, S., & Lebel, K. R. (2007). Crosslinguistic semantic and translation priming in normal bilingual individuals and bilingual aphasia. *Clinical Linguistics & Phonetics, 21*(4), 277–303.

Kirsner, K., Smith, M. C., Lockhart, R. S., King, M. L., & Jain, M. (1984). The bilingual lexicon: Language specific units in an integrated network. *Journal of Verbal Learning and Verbal Behavior, 23*, 519–539.

Kroll, J., & Curley, J. (1988). Lexical memory in novice bilinguals: The role of concepts in retrieving second language words. In M. Gruneberg, P. Morris, & R. Sykes (Eds.), *Practical aspects of memory* (Vol 2, pp. 389–395). London: John Wiley & Sons.

Kroll, J., & Stewart, E. (1994). Category interference in translation and picture naming: Evidence for asymmetric connections between bilingual memory representations. *Journal of Memory and Language, 33*, 149–174.

Kroll, J. F. K., & de Groot, A. M. B. (2005). *Handbook of bilingualism: Psycholinguistic approaches.* New York: Oxford University Press.

La Heij, W. (2005). Selection processes in monolingual and bilingual lexical access. In J. F. Kroll & A. M. B. de Groot (Eds.), *Handbook of bilingualism: Psycholinguistic approaches* (pp. 289–307). New York: Oxford University Press.

La Heij, W., de Bruyn, E., Elens, E., Hartsuiker, R., Helaha, D., & van Schelven, L. (1990). Orthographic facilitation and categorical interference in a word-translation variant of the Stroop task. *Canadian Journal of Psychology, 44*, 76–83.

La Heij, W., Hooglander, A., Kerling, R., & van der Velden, E. (1996). Nonverbal context effects in forward and backward word translation: Evidence for concept mediation. *Journal of Memory and Language, 35*, 648–665.

Laiacona, M., Barbarotto, R., Trivelli, C., & Capitani, E. (1993). Dissociazioni semantiche intercategoriali: descrizione di una batteria standardizzata e dati normativi. *Archivio di Psicologia, Neurologia e Psichiatria, 54*, 209–248.

Peña-Casanova, J. (2005). *Normalidad, semiología y patología neuropsicológicas. Programa integrado de exploración neuropsicológica. Test Barcelona Revisado (2°ed)*. Barcelona: Masson.

Poncelet, M., Majerus, S., Raman, I., Warginaire, S., & Weekes, B. S. (2007). Naming actions and objects in bilingual aphasia: A multiple case study. *Brain and Language, 103*, 158–159.

Potter, M. C., So, K. F., von Eckart, B., & Feldrnan, L. B. (1984). Lexical and conceptual representation in beginning and proficient bilinguals. *Journal of Verbal Learning and Verbal Behavior, 23*, 23–38.

Poulisse, N., & Bongaerts, T. (1994). First language use in second language production. *Applied Linguistics, 15*, 36–57.

Rami, L., Serradell, M., Bosch, B., Caprile, C., Sekler, A., Villar, A., et al. (2008). Normative data for the Boston Naming Test and the Pyramids and Palm Trees Test in the elderly Spanish population. *Journal of Clinical and Experimental Neuropsychology, 30*(1), 1–6.

Reisberg, B., Ferris, S. H., de León, M. J., & Crook, T. (1982). The global deterioration scale for assessment of primary degenerative dementia. *American Journal of Psychiatry, 139*, 1136–1139.

Riddoch, M. J., & Humphreys, G. W. (1993). *The Birmingham Object Recognition Battery (BORB)*. Hove, UK: Lawrence Erlbaum Associates Ltd.

Rodriguez-Fornells, A., van der Lugt, A., & Rotte, M. (2005). Second language interferes with word production in fluent bilinguals: Brain potential and functional imaging evidence. *Journal of Cognitive Neuroscience, 17*, 422–433.

Sanchez-Casas, R. M., Davis, C. W., & Garcia-Albea, J. E. (1992). Bilingual lexical processing: Exploring the cognate non-cognate distinction. *European Journal of Experimental Psychology, 4*(4), 293–310.

Sholl, A., Sankaranarayanan, A., & Kroll, J. F. (1995). Transfer between picture naming and translation: A test of asymmetries in bilingual memory. *Psychological Review, 96*, 523–568.

van Hell, J. G., & de Groot, A. M. B. (1998). Conceptual representation in bilingual memory: Effects of concreteness and cognate status in word association. *Bilingualism: Language and Cognition, 1*, 193–211.

van Hell, J. G., & Dijkstra, T. (2002). Foreign language knowledge can influence native language performance in exclusively native contexts. *Psychonomic Bulletin & Review, 9*, 780–789.

APPENDIX A: JFF'S LANGUAGE USE

JFF's first language was Catalan, but he started using Spanish before he started school (at the age of 7) with some distant relatives. Formal schooling was in Spanish (L2), a language that he also used with schoolmates. He used Catalan (L1) at home most of the time with his parents and siblings at first, and with his wife and daughter later. Although JFF left school at the age of 14 years, he kept using Spanish (L2) on a daily basis with some of his co-workers and friends at first, and with workers of his carpentry later.

JFF's bilingual profile was additionally reflected in a questionnaire filled out by his wife. This questionnaire generates language use scores, which reflect the frequency of use of each language in different stages of life and different contexts. The language use scores representing the amount of time JFF used his two languages (1 = *only Spanish*, 7 = *only Catalan*) are shown in the table below. JFF's language use scores reveal that he used to speak Catalan at home across his lifespan, while he mostly used Spanish at school. In addition, the frequency of use of both Catalan and Spanish across his lifespan was equivalent in places different from home and school, such as work and other social contexts. It is also worth mentioning that although

JFF's dominant language was clearly Catalan (L1), he was more proficient in L2 orthography relative to L1 due to the fact that he received formal education in Spanish but never in Catalan.

Finally, at the time of testing JFF only used Catalan (L1) on a daily basis because he only regularly interacted with his wife and daughter. Despite that, Spanish (L2) was not drastically affected relative to Catalan (L1) as shown by picture-naming results (see text).

	Preschool age	Childhood	Adolescence	Adulthood
School	–	3	–	–
Home	7	7	7	7
Other places	–	4	4	4

APPENDIX B: JFF'S NEUROPSYCHOLOGICAL PROFILE

JFF was diagnosed with AD in 1998 at the age of 74 years (7 years before testing him for the present study). At the moment of testing he was at a moderate-severe stage of the disease, measured by the Global Deterioration Scale (GDS; Reisberg, Ferris, de León, & Crook, 1982; JFF's GDS score = 5). JFF was unable to take care of his complex (e.g., to be in charge of the familiar economy, organising any activities, etc.) and instrumental (e.g., shopping, using phone, etc.) daily activities. He was highly dependent on his wife and needed supervision for his basic daily activities (e.g., dressing, personal hygiene, etc.). JFF was able to go out by himself only to very familiar places and always following the same route. He recognised close relatives and friends as well as habitual doctors and some acquaintances. JFF had accurate recall from youth; however, he had difficulties in encoding new information such as visitors from a few hours ago.

The cognitive screening carried out at the moment of testing by means of the Mini Mental State Examination (MMSE; Folstein, Folstein, & McHugh, 1975) evidenced a clear cognitive deterioration (JFF's MMSE score = 15). A more detailed neuropsychological examination was carried out by means of different subtests from the Spanish cognitive battery "Test Barcelona Revisado" (TBR; Peña-Casanova, 2005) which assesses different cognitive abilities. The TBR revealed personal, spatial, and temporal disorientation along with episodic memory impairment. JFF also had difficulties in imitating complex nonsense gestures and constructive praxes. His visuoconstructive ability was also impaired. JFF's spontaneous language was fluent and without grammatical errors. Although phonological or semantic errors were not present in spontaneous language, a pattern of semantic errors was observed in picture naming. Reading and writing and verbal repetition were preserved.

Additional examination on perceptual ability was carried out in order to rule out the possibility that poor results in naming were due to perceptual impairment. In particular, JFF's perceptual ability was assessed through the "overlapping figures" subtest of the Birmingham Object Recognition Battery (BORB; Riddoch & Humphreys, 1993). In this task JFF was asked to match stimuli of overlapping figures with the same non-overlapped stimuli. JFF's performance on this task was good: he obtained a score of 39 out of 40 correct responses; that is, he performed correctly on 97.5% of the items. This subtest of "overlapping figures" also served as a proof that JFF was able to perform well on some cognitive tasks despite his general cognitive impairment.

APPENDIX C: STIMULI FOR PICTURE NAMING AND TRANSLATION

The stimuli consisted of 62 items, half of which were cognates and the other half non-cognates. The same stimuli were used in L1 and L2 picture naming and in forward and backward translation.

Spanish and Catalan word frequency were not comparable due to the difference in the measures used by the Spanish and Catalan databases. Spanish and Catalan words were comparable in terms of length—Catalan: 5.61 phonemes, Spanish: 6.03 phonemes; $t(122) = 1.4$, $p = .16$.

Cognate and non-cognate stimuli were matched for Spanish lemma frequency (cognates: 11.7, non-cognates: 11.8) $t(60) = 0.03$, $p = .97$; Catalan lemma frequency (cognates: 633.6, non-cognates: 562.2) $t(60) = 0.41$, $p = .68$; Spanish familiarity (cognates: 3.4, non-cognates: 4.6) $t(60) = 1.5$, $p = .14$; Spanish imageability (cognates: 3.4, non-cognates: 4.5) $t(60) = 1.32$, $p = .19$; Spanish length (cognates: 6.3, non-cognates: 5.6) $t(60) = 1.16$, $p = .25$; and Catalan length (cognates: 5.71, non-cognates: 5.52) $t(60) = 0.48$, $p = .63$. No data are available on Catalan familiarity or imageability.

The criteria for considering a picture name as a cognate word were the following: (a) the Catalan and Spanish words for the picture share at least two consecutive phonemes in any position of the word, and/or (b) the Catalan and Spanish words for the picture share at least two phonemes in the same position of the word.

Cognate status of stimuli used in picture-naming and translation tasks

Cognates			Non-cognates		
Catalan name	Spanish name	English name	Catalan name	Spanish name	English name
Abella	Abeja	Bee	Mussol	Búho	Owl
Anell	Anillo	Ring	Mitjó	Calcetín	Sock
Cavall	Caballo	Horse	Raspall	Cepillo	Brush
Cacahuet	Cacahuete	Peanut	Estel	Cometa	Kite
Caixa	Caja	Box	Ganivet	Cuchillo	Knife
Carbassa	Calabaza	Pumpkin	Ulleres	Gafas	Glasses
Camell	Camello	Camel	Cuc	Gusano	Worm
Casc	Casco	Helmet	Destral	Hacha	Axe
Cirera	Cereza	Cherry	Enciam	Lechuga	Lettuce
Cèrvol	Ciervo	Deer	Clau anglesa	Llave inglesa	Spanner
Cinturó	Cinturón	Belt	Blat	Maíz	Corn
Clau	Clavo	Nail	Poma	Manzana	Apple
Cocodril	Cocodrilo	Crocodile	Papallona	Mariposa	Butterfly
Escombra	Escoba	Broom	Balancí	Mecedora	Rocking chair
Espàrrec	Espárrago	Asparagus	Préssec	Melocotón	Peach
Gat	Gato	Cat	Taronja	Naranja	Orange
Graner	Granero	Barn	Ocell	Pájaro	Bird
Guant	Guante	Glove	Ànec	Pato	Duck
Llagosta	Langosta	Lobster	Gos	Perro	Dog
Llapis	Lápiz	Pencil	Llit	Cama	Bed
Llimona	Limón	Lemon	Pebrot	Pimiento	Pepper
Molí	Molino	Windmill	Granota	Rana	Frog
Nas	Nariz	Nose	Paella	Sartén	Frying Pan
Núvol	Nube	Cloud	Bolet	Seta	Mushroom
Ovella	Oveja	Sheep	Xiulet	Silbato	Whistle
Pantalons	Pantalones	Trousers	Cadira	Silla	Chair
Pilota	Pelota	Ball	Barret	Sombrero	Hat
Rinoceront	Rinoceronte	Rhinoceros	Forquilla	Tenedor	Fork
Saler	Salero	Salt shaker	Raïm	Uva	Grapes
Tomàquet	Tomate	Tomato	Pastanaga	Zanahoria	Carrot
Violí	Violín	Violin	Guineu	Zorro	Fox

APPENDIX D: JFF'S ERROR TRANSCRIPTION AND CLASSIFICATION

JFF's errors are organised by items and broken down by task (✓=Correct response from JFF). Errors were classified into three types: semantic (SEM), inappropriate word forms (IWF), and non-responses (NR) (see Results section).

	Correct response	Transcription of JFF's errors	English translation of JFF's errors	Error type
English name: OWL				
NAMING L1	Mussol	Un àguila petita.	A small eagle.	SEM
NAMING L2	Búho	Esto es un pájaro, pero no sé qué pájaro es esto.	It's a bird, but I don't know what type of bird it is.	SEM
FORWARD TRANSLATION (L1→L2)	Búho	Mussuelo.	(stem of L1 word inflection)	IWF
BACKWARD TRANSLATION (L2→L1)	Mussol	Això diria que és el nom d'una bèstia. Ara no sé com li diuen …	I'd say that it's the name of an animal. I don't know what it's called …	SEM
English name: SOCK				
NAMING L1	Mitjó	✓		
NAMING L2	Calcetín	✓		
FORWARD TRANSLATION (L1→L2)	Calcetín	Michón.	(stem of L1 word inflection)	IWF
BACKWARD TRANSLATION (L2→L1)	Mitjó	✓		
English name: BRUSH				
NAMING L1	Raspall	✓		
NAMING L2	Cepillo	Un raspallo.	(L1 word inflection)	IWF
FORWARD TRANSLATION (L1→L2)	Cepillo	Respaldo.	(stem of L1 word inflection that resulted in a existing word [back])	IWF
BACKWARD TRANSLATION (L2→L1)	Raspall	Un cepillo es un fregador.	(semantically related noun + inflection)	SEM
English name: KITE				
NAMING L1	Estel	Un juguet de volar	A flying toy.	SEM
NAMING L2	Cometa	Esto es para volar, para atar así y volar.	It's for flying; it is for tying like that and flying.	SEM
FORWARD TRANSLATION (L1→L2)	Cometa	Estelo.	(stem of L1 word inflection)	IWF
BACKWARD TRANSLATION (L2→L1)	Estel	Una c/u/méta	(regularisation of the L2 non-cognate word as if it was a cognate one)	IWF

	Correct response	Transcription of JFF's errors	English translation of JFF's errors	Error type
English name: LETTUCE				
NAMING L1	Enciam	Sembla una taronja. Però pot ser una altra classe de fruita. Hi ha cols que semblen aixi.	It looks like an orange. But it may be another type of fruit. Some cabbages look like that.	SEM
NAMING L2	Lechuga	Parece una planta, parece como ... una naranja. No, una naranja no, una pera.	It looks like a plant; it looks like ... an orange. No, not an orange, a pear.	SEM
FORWARD TRANSLATION (L1→L2)	Lechuga	✓		
BACKWARD TRANSLATION (L2→L1)	Enciam	Una verdura	A vegetable	SEM
English name: WORM				
NAMING L1	Cuc	✓		
NAMING L2	Gusano	No sabría decir esto qué es.	I can't tell what that is	NR
FORWARD TRANSLATION (L1→L2)	Gusano	Cuco.	(stem of L1 word inflection)	IWF
BACKWARD TRANSLATION (L2→L1)	Cuc	Tant en Català com en Castellà podria ser un gos.	It might be a dog both in Catalan and Spanish.	SEM
English name: AXE				
NAMING L1	Destral	✓		
NAMING L2	Hacha	✓		
FORWARD TRANSLATION (L1→L2)	Hacha	També es diuen destral.	(L1 word)	IWF
BACKWARD TRANSLATION (L2→L1)	Destral	✓		
English name: CORN				
NAMING L1	Blat	Això sembla algo dels arbres.	It seems like something having to do with trees.	SEM
NAMING L2	Maíz	Esto es una fruta que ...¿Cómo se llama? No un plátano porque tiene piezas por dentro.	It's a fruit that ... What's its name? It isn't a banana because it has pieces inside.	SEM
FORWARD TRANSLATION (L1→L2)	Maíz	...	...	NR
BACKWARD TRANSLATION (L2→L1)	Blat	Per menjar ...	To eat ...	SEM
English name: APPLE				
NAMING L1	Poma	Això és una poma. No! Això és una pera.	This is an apple. No! This is a pear.	SEM
NAMING L2	Manzana	✓		
FORWARD TRANSLATION (L1→L2)	Manzana	Poma també.	(L1 word)	IWF
BACKWARD TRANSLATION (L2→L1)	Poma	És una taronja. Ai! És una mandarina.	It's an orange. Oh! A mandarine	SEM

	Correct response	Transcription of JFF's errors	English translation of JFF's errors	Error type
English name: BUTTERFLY				
NAMING L1	Papallona	✓		
NAMING L2	Mariposa	Esto vuela …	It flies …	SEM
FORWARD TRANSLATION (L1→L2)	Papallona	Una papallona.	(L1 word)	IWF
BACKWARD TRANSLATION (L2→L1)	Mariposa	✓		
English name: ROCKING CHAIR				
NAMING L1	Balancí	Una cadira de groxar-se.	A chair for rocking.	SEM
NAMING L2	Mecedora	La silla para groncharte tú mismo.	The chair for rocking (Catalan verb inflection) oneself.	SEM
FORWARD TRANSLATION (L1→L2)	Mecedora	Una siesta.	A nap	SEM
BACKWARD TRANSLATION (L2→L1)	Balancí	Una mesa.	A table.	SEM
English name: PEACH				
NAMING L1	Préssec	Sembla una fruita.	It looks like a fruit.	SEM
NAMING L2	Melocotón	No sé qué podría ser esto …	I don't know what it might be …	NR
FORWARD TRANSLATION (L1→L2)	Melocotón	✓		
BACKWARD TRANSLATION (L2→L1)	Préssec	Meló.	A watermelon.	SEM
English name: ORANGE				
NAMING L1	Taronja	Sembla … les pomes, també les taronges …	It seems … apples, also oranges …	SEM
NAMING L2	Naranjna	✓		
FORWARD TRANSLATION (L1→L2)	Naranja	✓		
BACKWARD TRANSLATION (L2→L1)	Taronja	✓		
English name: DUCK				
NAMING L1	Ànec	Una gosseta.	A little dog.	SEM
NAMING L2	Pato	Una bestia pero no sé el nombre que es.	An animal but I don't know its name.	SEM
FORWARD TRANSLATION (L1→L2)	Pato	Una hembra porque tiene alas.	A female because it has wings. (stem of L1 word inflection)	IWF
BACKWARD TRANSLATION (L2→L1)	Ànec	Ánago.	…	NR

	Correct response	Transcription of JFF's errors	English translation of JFF's errors	Error type
English name: BED				
NAMING L1	Llit	✓		
NAMING L2	Cama	✓		
FORWARD TRANSLATION (L1→L2)	Cama	Cama també.	(L1 word)	IWF
BACKWARD TRANSLATION (L2→L1)	Llit	✓		
English name: PEPPER				
NAMING L1	Pebrot	Sembla una pera.	It looks like a pear.	SEM
NAMING L2	Pimiento	Una fruta …	A fruit …	SEM
FORWARD TRANSLATION (L1→L2)	Pimiento	Pebrote.	(stem of L1 word inflection)	IWF
BACKWARD TRANSLATION (L2→L1)	Pebrot	Diria que és una poma.	I'd say it's an apple.	SEM
English name: FROG				
NAMING L1	Granota	Aquestes bèsties que salten.	Those animals that jump.	SEM
NAMING L2	Rana	Ahora no sé si es una tortuga o es una oruga. ¿Cómo le llaman a estas que saltan?	I don't know whether it's a turtle or a worm. What do you call those animals that jump? (Imitation of the frog sound).	SEM
FORWARD TRANSLATION (L1→L2)	Rana	Granota.	(L1 word)	IWF
BACKWARD TRANSLATION (L2→L1)	Granota	✓		
English name: FRYING PAN				
NAMING L1	Paella	Una garrafa.	A bottle.	SEM
NAMING L2	Sartén	Paella també.	(L1 name).	IWF
FORWARD TRANSLATION (L1→L2)	Sartén	Una paja.	(stem of L1 word inflection that resulted in a existing word [back])	IWF
BACKWARD TRANSLATION (L2→L1)	Paella	✓		
English name: MUSHROOM				
NAMING L1	Bolet	✓		
NAMING L2	Seta	… en Castellano … un bolet? Una cebolla.	… in Spanish … (L1 name)? An onion.	SEM
FORWARD TRANSLATION (L1→L2)	Seta	Boleto.	(stem of L1 word inflection)	IWF
BACKWARD TRANSLATION (L2→L1)	Bolet	Per menjar …	To eat …	SEM

	Correct response	Transcription of JFF's errors	English translation of JFF's errors	Error type
English name: WHISTLE				
NAMING L1	Xiulet	✓		
NAMING L2	Silbato	No sé qué es ...	I don't know what that is ...	NR
FORWARD TRANSLATION (L1→L2)	Silbato	Un silbido.	(stem of L2 word inflection that resulted in a existing word [whistling])	SEM
BACKWARD TRANSLATION (L2→L1)	Xiulet	✓		
English name: FORK				
NAMING L1	Forquilla	✓		
NAMING L2	Tenedor	Una orquilla. En Castellano forquilla es orquilla, no?	(L1 word form without the first phoneme).	IWF
FORWARD TRANSLATION (L1→L2)	Tenedor	Orquilla.	(L1 word form without the first phoneme)	IWF
BACKWARD TRANSLATION (L2→L1)	Forquilla	Una cullera.	A spoon.	SEM
English name: CHAIR				
NAMING L1	Cadira	Una cosa per seure la gent.	A thing for people to sit.	SEM
NAMING L2	Silla	✓		
FORWARD TRANSLATION (L1→L2)	Silla	✓		
BACKWARD TRANSLATION (L2→L1)	Cadira	✓		
English name: GRAPES				
NAMING L1	Raïm	Això sembla les taronges ... això sembla allò que mengem per postres. Una branqueta de pinyons.	It looks like oranges ... it looks like that dessert we eat ... A little branch of pine nuts.	SEM
NAMING L2	Uva	Cerezas.	Cherries.	SEM
FORWARD TRANSLATION (L1→L2)	Uva	✓		
BACKWARD TRANSLATION (L2→L1)	Raïm	✓		
English name: CARROT				
NAMING L1	Pastanaga	Una fruita ...	A fruit ...	SEM
NAMING L2	Zanahoria	Eso de comer ...	We eat that ...	SEM
FORWARD TRANSLATION (L1→L2)	Zanahoria	Pastanaga també.	(L1 word)	IWF
BACKWARD TRANSLATION (L2→L1)	Pastanaga	Una ceba.	An onion.	SEM

	Correct response	Transcription of JFF's errors	English translation of JFF's errors	Error type
English name: FOX				
NAMING L1	Guineu	Una pantera.	A panther.	SEM
NAMING L2	Zorro	Eso es una perra.	This is a [female] dog.	SEM
FORWARD TRANSLATION (L1→L2)	Zorro	Guinéo.	(stem of L1 word inflection)	IWF
BACKWARD TRANSLATION (L2→L1)	Guineu	Una ... serp, no?	A ... snake, right?	SEM
English name: BEE				
NAMING L1	Abella	Una bestieta.	A little animal	SEM
NAMING L2	Abeja	Esto es una bestia ... ¿Cómo le llaman? Son bestias pequeñas.	This is an animal ... What is it called? They are little animals.	SEM
FORWARD TRANSLATION (L1→L2)	Abeja	Oveja	(L2 phonological error that resulted in a SEM existing word [sheep])	
BACKWARD TRANSLATION (L2→L1)	Abella	✓		
English name: RING				
NAMING L1	Anell	No sabria dir què és això.	I don't know what to say.	NR
NAMING L2	Anillo	Esto sí que no sé qué es.	I don't know what that is.	NR
FORWARD TRANSLATION (L1→L2)	Anillo	✓		
BACKWARD TRANSLATION (L2→L1)	Anell	✓		
English name: HORSE				
NAMING L1	Cavall	Una gossa o un gos, és igual. Una ternera, o ... bueno, és una bèstia.	A [female] dog or a dog, it doesn't matter. A calf, or ... OK, it's an animal.	SEM
NAMING L2	Caballo	✓		
FORWARD TRANSLATION (L1→L2)	Caballo	✓		
BACKWARD TRANSLATION (L2→L1)	Cavall	✓		
English name: PEANUT				
NAMING L1	Cacahuet	No sé qué és ...	I don't know what it is ...	NR
NAMING L2	Cacahuete	No sé esto qué podría ser ...	I don't know what it could be ...	NR
FORWARD TRANSLATION (L1→L2)	Cacahuete	✓		
BACKWARD TRANSLATION (L2→L1)	Cacahuet	✓		

	Correct response	Transcription of JFF's errors	English translation of JFF's errors	Error type
English name: BOX				
NAMING L1	Capsa	✓		
NAMING L2	Caja	Una bolsa para poner cosas dentro.	A bag to put things in.	SEM
FORWARD TRANSLATION (L1 → L2)	Caja	✓		
BACKWARD TRANSLATION (L2 → L1)	Capsa	✓		
English name: PUMPKIN				
NAMING L1	Carbassa	No sé què dir ...	I don't know what to say ...	NR
NAMING L2	Calabaza	No sé ... esto ...	I don't know ... it ...	NR
FORWARD TRANSLATION (L1 → L2)	Calabaza	✓		
BACKWARD TRANSLATION (L2 → L1)	Carbassa	✓		
English name: CAMEL				
NAMING L1	Camell	... aquestes bèsties. Els que tenen aquest bony aquí dalt tenen un altre nom ...	... those animals. The ones that have this lump up here have a different name ...	SEM
NAMING L2	Camello	Esto es una bestia pero no sé el nombre. Es una bestia de las playas. Ay! No de las playas ... de los sitios que vamos a ver.	It's an animal but I don't know its name. It's an animal from the beach ... Oh! Not from the beach ... from places we go to visit.	SEM
FORWARD TRANSLATION (L1 → L2)	Camello	✓		
BACKWARD TRANSLATION (L2 → L1)	Camell	✓		
English name: HELMET				
NAMING L1	Casc	No sé què és ... sembla ...	I don't know what it is ... it seems ...	NR
NAMING L2	Casco	Nunca he visto algo como esto.	I've never seen anything like that.	NR
FORWARD TRANSLATION (L1 → L2)	Casc	✓		
BACKWARD TRANSLATION (L2 → L1)	Casco	Un sombrero.	A hat.	SEM
English name: CHERRY				
NAMING L1	Cirera	Una poma.	An apple.	SEM
NAMING L2	Cereza	Una manzana.	An apple.	SEM
FORWARD TRANSLATION (L1 → L2)	Cereza	✓		
BACKWARD TRANSLATION (L2 → L1)	Cirera	✓		

	Correct response	Transcription of JFF's errors	English translation of JFF's errors	Error type
English name: DEER				
NAMING L1	Cérvol	... hi ha les tortugues ... té un nom això ...	... there are the turtles ... it has a name ...	SEM
NAMING L2	Ciervo	Esto no sé el nombre ..., una tortuga ... no, ...	I don't know its name ... a turtle ... no ...	SEM
FORWARD TRANSLATION (L1 → L2)	Ciervo	Siérvol.	(L1 word form + wrong phoneme)	IWF
BACKWARD TRANSLATION (L2 → L1)	Cérvol	...	...	NR
English name: BROOM				
NAMING L1	Escombra	Una alfombra per escombrar.	A carpet to sweep.	SEM
NAMING L2	Escoba	✓		
FORWARD TRANSLATION (L1 → L2)	Escoba	✓		
BACKWARD TRANSLATION (L2 → L1)	Escombra	✓		
English name: NAIL				
NAMING L1	Clau	✓		
NAMING L2	Clavo	Un eso para atornillar ...	That thing to screw things down ...	SEM
FORWARD TRANSLATION (L1 → L2)	Clavo	✓		
BACKWARD TRANSLATION (L2 → L1)	Clau	✓		
English name: CROCODILE				
NAMING L1	Cocodril	✓		
NAMING L2	Cocodrilo	Una dragona pequeña.	A little dragon.	SEM
FORWARD TRANSLATION (L1 → L2)	Cocodrilo	C/u/c/u/drilo.	(L1 phonology)	IWF
BACKWARD TRANSLATION (L2 → L1)	Cocodril	✓		
English name: ASPARAGUS				
NAMING L1	Espàrrec	Això si que no sé el nom.	I don't know the name of it.	NR
NAMING L2	Espárrago	Una branca.	A branch (L1)	SEM
FORWARD TRANSLATION (L1 → L2)	Espárrago	Lagosta.	(mix of L1 and L2 phonology)	IWF
BACKWARD TRANSLATION (L2 → L1)	Espàrrec	✓		

	Correct response	Transcription of JFF's errors	English translation of JFF's errors	Error type
English name: CAT				
NAMING L1	Gat	✓		
NAMING L2	Gato	Esto es una bestia pero no sé el nombre, porque no es un gato ni nada de eso.	This is an animal but I don't know its name, because it isn't a cat or anything like that.	SEM
FORWARD TRANSLATION (L1→L2)	Gato	✓		
BACKWARD TRANSLATION (L2→L1)	Gat	✓		
English name: BARN				
NAMING L1	Graner	No sé el nom ...	I don't know the name ...	NR
NAMING L2	Granero	No sé qué es ...	I don't know what that is ...	NR
FORWARD TRANSLATION (L1→L2)	Granero	✓		
BACKWARD TRANSLATION (L2→L1)	Graner	Això si que no sé què és.	I don't know what that is.	NR
English name: GLOVE				
NAMING L1	Guant	Sembla ...	It seems ...	NR
NAMING L2	Guante	No sé esto qué podría ser.	I don't know what it could be.	NR
FORWARD TRANSLATION (L1→L2)	Guante	✓		
BACKWARD TRANSLATION (L2→L1)	Guant	✓		
English name: LOBSTER				
NAMING L1	Llagosta	Això és una bèstia del mar.	This is an animal from the sea.	SEM
NAMING L2	Langosta	Una bestia. Sé que la he visto a veces en el Parque.	An animal. I know I've seen it in the zoo.	SEM
FORWARD TRANSLATION (L1→L2)	Langosta	✓		
BACKWARD TRANSLATION (L2→L1)	Llagosta	✓		
English name: LEMON				
NAMING L1	Llimona	Sembla una taronja ... és com una mandarina, però té un altre nom ...	It looks like an orange ... it's like a mandarin, but it has a different name ...	SEM
NAMING L2	Limón	Esto parece una naranja. Ay! No, una naranja no ...	It seems like an orange. No! Not an orange ...	SEM
FORWARD TRANSLATION (L1→L2)	Limón	✓		
BACKWARD TRANSLATION (L2→L1)	Llimona	✓		

	Correct response	Transcription of JFF's errors	English translation of JFF's errors	Error type
English name: WINDMILL				
NAMING L1	Molí	No sé qué és ...	I don't know what it is ...	NR
NAMING L2	Molino	Un ventilador. Ay! No un ventilador. Hay casas que hay esto ... en el campo.	A fan. No! Not a fan. Some houses have that ... in the country.	SEM
FORWARD TRANSLATION (L1→L2)	Molino	✓		
BACKWARD TRANSLATION (L2→L1)	Molí	✓		
English name: CLOUD				
NAMING L1	Núvol	✓		
NAMING L2	Nube	No sé qué es ...	I don't know what that is ...	NR
FORWARD TRANSLATION (L1→L2)	Nube	Núvulo	(L1 word+inflection)	IWF
BACKWARD TRANSLATION (L2→L1)	Núvol	✓		
English name: SHEEP				
NAMING L1	Ovella	Això és ... com li diuen a aquestes bèsties? Això és un mascle perquè a les femelles se li veu ... una tortuga. Ai no! Una tortuga no ...	This is ... what do they call those animals? This is a male because in females you can see ... a turtle. Oh no! Not a turtle ...	SEM
NAMING L2	Oveja	Esto parece una perra. Espere! ...	It looks like a [female] dog. Wait! ...	SEM
FORWARD TRANSLATION (L1→L2)	Oveja	✓		
BACKWARD TRANSLATION (L2→L1)	Ovella	Papallones.	Butterflies	SEM
English name: RHINOCEROS				
NAMING L1	Rinoceront	Com li diuen a aquesta bèstia que porta això?	What do they call that animal that has this thing?	SEM
NAMING L2	Rinoceronte	No sé qué decir si una perra o un perro ...	I'm not sure whether it's a [female] dog or a [male] dog ...	SEM
FORWARD TRANSLATION (L1→L2)	Rinoceronte	✓		
BACKWARD TRANSLATION (L2→L1)	Rinoceront	✓		

	Correct response	Transcription of JFF's errors	English translation of JFF's errors	Error type
English name: SALT SHAKER				
NAMING L1	Saler	Sembla ...	It looks like ...	NR
NAMING L2	Salero	Una copa.	A glass.	SEM
FORWARD TRANSLATION (L1 → L2)	Salero	... jo diria saler.	(L1 word)	IWF
BACKWARD TRANSLATION (L2 → L1)	Saler	✓		
English name: TOMATO				
NAMING L1	Tomàquet	Pot ser una poma ... però pot ser una altra fruita també ...	It may be an apple ... but it may also be another type of fruit ...	SEM
NAMING L2	Tomate	Es una lechuga. Una mandarina.	It's lettuce. It's a mandarine.	SEM
FORWARD TRANSLATION (L1 → L2)	Tomate	Una pimienta.	A pepper	SEM
BACKWARD TRANSLATION (L2 → L1)	Tomàquet	✓		
English name: VIOLIN				
NAMING L1	Violí	✓		
NAMING L2	Violín	Es un eso para tocar música.	It's a thing to play music.	SEM
FORWARD TRANSLATION (L1 → L2)	Violín	✓		
BACKWARD TRANSLATION (L2 → L1)	Violí	Un violó	(L2 stem + phonological error)	IWF

APHASIOLOGY, 2010, 24 (2), 170–187

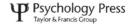

Cross-language treatment generalisation: A case of trilingual aphasia

Mira Goral

Lehman College, The City University of New York, NY, USA

Erika S. Levy and Rebecca Kastl

Teachers College, Columbia University, NY, USA

Background: Recent investigations of language gains following treatment in bilingual individuals with chronic aphasia appear to confirm early reports that not only the treated language but also the non-treated language(s) benefit from treatment. The evidence, however, is still suggestive, and the variables that may mitigate generalisation across languages warrant further investigation.

Aims: We set out to examine cross-language generalisation of language treatment in a trilingual speaker with mild chronic aphasia.

Methods & Procedures: Language treatment was administered in English, the participant's second language (L2). The first treatment block focused on morphosyntactic skills and the second on language production rate. Measurements were collected in the treated language (English, L2) as well as the two non-treated languages: Hebrew (the participant's first language, L1) and French (the participant's third language, L3).

Outcomes & Results: The participant showed improvement in his production of selected morphosyntactic elements, such as pronoun gender agreement, in the treated language (L2) as well as in the non-treated French (L3) following the treatment block that focused on morphosyntactic skills. Speech rate also improved in English (L2) and French (L3) following that treatment block. No changes were observed in Hebrew, the participant's L1.

Conclusions: Selective cross-language generalisation of treatment benefit was found for morphosyntactic abilities from the participant's second language to his third language.

Keywords: Aphasia; Trilingual; Treatment; Cross-language generalisation; Morphosyntax.

Recent investigations of gains following language treatment in bilingual individuals with aphasia (e.g., Edmonds & Kiran, 2006) are consistent with early reports (e.g., Paradis, 1993; Watamori & Sasanuma, 1978) that not only the treated language but

Address correspondence to: Mira Goral PhD, CCC-SLP, Associate Professor, Speech-Language-Hearing Sciences, Lehman College, 250 Bedford Park Blvd. Bronx, NY 10468, USA. E-mail: mira.goral@lehman.cuny.edu

We thank Eyal Cohen for his participation in this study and for his insights. We also thank Catharine Castellucio, Niri Halperin, Natalia Martínez, Keren Ohayon, and Tali Swann-Sternberg for their assistance with data coding, and Daniel Kempler for numerous discussions. We thank the editor, Brendan Weekes for his support, and two anonymous reviewers for their helpful comments. Support for this research was provided to Mira Goral by NIH grants AG27532-01A1 and GM081113-01.

http://www.psypress.com/aphasiology   DOI: 10.1080/02687030902958308

also the non-treated language(s) benefit from intervention. However, the evidence is still suggestive, and the variables that may mitigate generalisation across languages warrant further investigation.

Cross-language treatment generalisation may depend on the status of the treated language; that is, whether the treatment is provided in the person's first language (L1) versus the second language (L2) or in the dominant language versus the less-dominant language. For example, Edmonds and Kiran (2006) found cross-language generalisation only when the non-treated language was the speaker's more dominant language or when the participants were highly proficient in both their languages. Edmonds and Kiran administered naming treatment to two bilingual individuals. Their first participant, who was dominant in English and less proficient in Spanish, demonstrated improvement only in the treated language when treated in his dominant language (English), and improvement in both the treated and the non-treated languages when treated in his less dominant language (Spanish). Their second participant was a balanced bilingual. He was treated in Spanish only and demonstrated improvement in both the treated and the non-treated languages. The authors attributed this difference in their participants' response to treatment to the difference in their dominance level of the non-treated languages.

Studies have also shown that cross-language generalisation might be limited to those linguistic aspects that are common to the two languages under investigation. For example, Kohnert (2004) found differential results for cognates (i.e., translation equivalents that share their meaning and form) as compared to non-cognates (i.e., translation equivalents that share their meaning but differ in form). These results are consistent with the unique role of cognates in the bilingual lexicon (e.g., Lalor & Kirsner, 2001). Furthermore, specific characteristics of the language components being treated might determine the patterns of impairment and recovery observed in each language. For example, Ullman and his colleagues (e.g., Ullman, 2006; Ullman et al., 2005) have proposed that syntactic aspects, hypothesised to be acquired implicitly (via procedural memory) in L1 but explicitly (via declarative memory) in L2 and other non-L1 languages (at least for late learners), are likely to have independent representation in the two languages. In contrast, the lexicon, hypothesised to be part of the declarative memory system in L1 as well as in L2 and other non-L1 languages, is suggested to have greater overlap in the two languages. An increasing amount of clinical and neuroimaging data supports the distinction and the localisation of the two memory systems in distinct neural networks (e.g., Friederici, 2004; Friederici, Hahne, & von Cramon, 1998; Ullman et al., 2005).

It is reasonable to assume that the representation and processing of linguistic aspects that are common to two languages would overlap more than the representation and processing of aspects that differ across languages and would thus potentially facilitate cross-language generalisation. Moreover, neuroimaging data from bilingual speakers suggest overlapping systems for the two languages of highly proficient bilinguals (e.g., Chee, Tan, & Thiel, 1999; Perani & Abutalebi, 2005). Further discussion of language representation and processing in the multilingual brain is beyond the scope of this paper (for reviews see Abutalebi, Cappa, & Perani, 2001; Abutalebi & Green, 2007; Paradis, 2004; Roberts, 2008; Vaid & Hull, 2002), yet assumptions concerning the dissociation between separate and shared representations in the languages of bilingual and multilingual individuals could yield predictions regarding cross-language generalisation, and guide clinicians' choices about which language to treat.

The question of which language to treat has received little mention in the research literature (e.g., Gil & Goral, 2004; Paradis, 1983). From a clinical standpoint, bilingual individuals who have aphasia ought to receive treatment in any and all their languages, but this is rarely feasible. For many bilingual individuals who live in their L2 environment, speech-language treatment is often available only in their L2. This is true for many individuals living in countries in which the primary language(s) spoken is not their first language, including, for example, the United States (e.g., Levy et al., 2007; Wiener, Obler, Taylor-Sarno, 1995), the UK and Scotland (e.g., Mennen & Stansfield, 2006; Winter, 1999), Australia (e.g., Diaz, 2003), and East Africa (e.g., Jochmann, 2006). Therefore it is critical to determine whether treating individuals' L2 can yield positive outcomes in their L1 (or any other languages they speak) and if so, what language components are most likely to benefit from treatment. This information is required for the appropriate selection of the language or languages of treatment.

In the present study we employed a within-participant design to examine cross-language generalisation in aphasia treatment. We enrolled a trilingual speaker with aphasia, administered language treatment in English (L2), and tested his three languages pre- and post-treatment. We predicted that the participant would show treatment-related gains in the skills addressed in the treated language (his L2). In addition, we predicted that if languages of high proficiency are represented and processed in largely overlapping neural networks, we should observe cross-language generalisation for treatment gains to the participant's non-treated L1 (Hebrew) and L3 (French). If, however, language status (i.e., being the first- versus later-acquired language, being the more- or less-proficient language) affects language representation and therefore the occurrence of cross-language treatment generalisation, differential patterns would be detected for the non-treated L1 (Hebrew) versus the non-treated L3 (French).

METHOD

Case details

EC, a 49-year-old right-handed trilingual Hebrew–English–French speaker with chronic mild nonfluent aphasia participated in this study. Prior to his stroke EC had completed a doctorate and post-doctoral work in physics, and worked as the director of a computer animation company he founded. EC has not returned to work since his stroke. EC's first language was Hebrew, acquired from birth. He achieved native-like proficiency in Hebrew and used it extensively as a young adult and infrequently during the decade prior to his aphasia onset. His second language was English. He was exposed to English in infancy, as he was born in the US (although to Hebrew-speaking parents). After moving to Israel at age 3, he did not speak or hear English until he began learning it formally at school at the age of 10. Starting in his early 20s he began using English extensively while pursuing his higher education and later working in the US in the years prior to the aphasia onset. French was his third language, learned formally beginning at 16 and then used extensively during his post-doctoral studies and work in France, where he lived for approximately 15 years. At the time of the aphasia onset, French was the language used at home for communication among EC's family members. Reportedly, EC had achieved very high proficiency in all modalities in these three languages. In addition he enjoyed

TABLE 1
Summary of EC's language history

	L1	L2	L3
Language	Hebrew	English	French
Age learned	Birth	Age 10	Age 16
How learned	Acquired at home	Exposed in infancy; learned formally; then by immersion	Learned formally; then by immersion
Language use at the time of aphasia onset	Rarely (with extended family)	Frequently (at work, with friends, in the environment)	Frequently (with immediate family at home)
Proficiency	High	High	High
Language use at time of treatment	Frequently (for practice)	Frequently (in the environment; for practice)	Frequently (with family; for practice)
Language of treatment	Non-treated language	Treated language	Non-treated language

learning languages and had working knowledge of Spanish, German, and Italian. For a summary of EC's language history, see Table 1.

At age 42, EC experienced a left MCA CVA, resulting in a large fronto-temporo-parietal lesion. In the 6 months immediately following his stroke, he experienced right hemiplegia and severe deficits in all languages. With time, his right-sided weakness resolved and he demonstrated steady improvement in his three languages. According to self-report, confirmed by our pre-treatment testing using the Bilingual Aphasia Battery (BAT, Paradis & Libben, 1987; see Figure 1), his Hebrew recovered better than the other two languages (despite infrequent use for a decade pre-onset) and his French recovered least (despite high proficiency and frequent use). (For additional information about EC's abilities in his three languages see Goral, Levy, Obler, & Cohen, 2006.)

Prior to the treatment provided in the course of the current study EC had received individual treatment in English for 5 months immediately following his stroke. About 1 year following his stroke he started to attend an aphasia support group, in which he continues to participate twice a week. At the time of the study, EC had been using the computer for email exchanges and Internet browsing, listening to books on tapes, and using a variety of workbooks in his three languages. He demonstrated high motivation and dedication to improving his language abilities.

At the time the study began, 7 years post-onset, EC experienced mild aphasia, no hemiplegia, and no dysarthria. Informal assessment revealed no perceptual or cognitive impairment. His language comprehension was nearly intact. His oral language production was characterised by slow rate and frequent hesitations and rephrasing. He produced mostly complete sentences, but these were filled with false starts, self-corrections, and some uncorrected grammatical errors. His word-finding abilities were good in isolation but he experienced word-finding difficulties during connected speech production.

Treatment design and details

Treatment. Treatment was conducted in EC's L2, English, by a native speaker of English. Therapy consisted of two 3-week periods of nine 1-hour sessions each with a

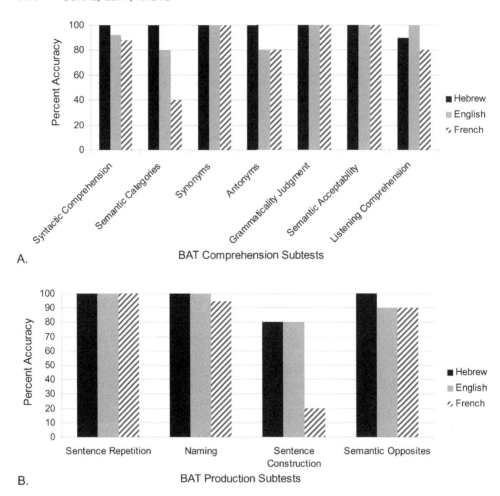

Figure 1. Percent accuracy on the Bilingual Aphasia Test (BAT) Comprehension Subtests (A) and Production Subtests (B).

break of 3 weeks with no treatment in between. We administered treatments with two different foci. The first treatment targeted morphosyntactic constructions (e.g., tense consistency, pronoun agreement, noun–verb agreement). The second treatment targeted language production rate. The treatment activities were similar in both treatment blocks and included a number of barrier activities, structured conversation, and verbal description of pictures. Because of EC's good comprehension skills and adequate production skills at the word and phrase level, our treatment focused on language production in sentence and discourse context. Furthermore, our approach to treatment emphasised informative exchanges between EC and the clinician. That is, our goal was to minimise drill-based exercises and maximise language production in meaningful contexts (e.g., Goral & Kempler, in press; Meinzer, Elbert, Djundja, Taub, & Rockstruh, 2007). To this end, in both treatment blocks we used an array of pictures or verbal stimuli, and a barrier. For each exchange, EC was instructed to select a stimulus (e.g., a photograph of a painting) and to produce connected speech to describe it. The clinician, in turn, tried to guess what stimulus was being described. For each array of stimuli, a range of responses (e.g., different descriptions of paintings) was acceptable. Therefore, EC's production was required to be informative in order for the clinician to be able to identify the selected stimulus. Typically, EC produced sufficient information for the exchange to be successful. When needed, however, the clinician clarified EC's utterance, modelling a complete and correct response. In the course of the session, EC and the clinician took turns describing stimuli and exchanging information.

The difference between the two treatment periods was primarily in the type of feedback and correction provided by the clinician. In the first treatment block (morphosyntax), the clinician corrected any morphosyntactic error that EC produced and modelled correct production. The clinician and EC engaged in explicit discussions of sentence structure, morphological rules, etc. For example, EC was instructed to select a picture from an array of two to five pictures and to describe it to the clinician. The clinician identified the picture that EC was describing, provided him with feedback about the grammaticality of his production, modelled the correct structures, and elicited EC's correct production. In the second treatment block (language production rate), materials and tasks similar to those used in the first treatment block were employed. During this block, however, the clinician did not address EC's grammatical and morphosyntactic errors but focused instead on proceeding with his sentence. She encouraged him to employ word-finding strategies, such as circumlocutions, and to continue with his sentence production, even if the target word was not successfully retrieved and if grammatical errors were produced. For example, EC was again instructed to select a picture from an array and describe it as fluently as he could. The clinician identified the picture that EC described and then provided feedback concerning his language production rate, word-retrieval rate, and his use of strategies to avoid long pauses.

We note that the treatment sessions included explicit discussion of morphosyntactic rules, language structures, and strategies. As such, the treatment not only provided EC with the opportunity to practise his language production skills but also addressed metalinguistic abilities.

Because the participant lived in California and the Hebrew–English and French–English bilingual researchers were in New York,[1] we implemented long-distance testing and therapy over the computer using Skype[TM]. The (student) clinician (the third author) used a sound-treated booth at the Speech Production and Perception Lab at Teachers College, Columbia University. The participant used his home desktop computer. He and the clinician saw each other on the computer (Dell[TM] Optiplex GX520 Desktop Computer) screen using cameras (Logitech Quickcam[©] Pro 5000 webcam), and heard each other using headphones. Appointments were scheduled for the duration of the treatment and any materials needed were sent prior to the treatment period. The materials included packets of duplicated numbered picture stimuli so that EC and the clinician could refer to the same series of stimuli.

---

[1] At this time post stroke, EC is no longer eligible for medically covered speech-language treatment. However, he has remained highly motivated and interested in working on his language skills and maintaining his multilingualism. He had expressed interest to the first author in participating in a treatment study that would focus on multilingual individuals with aphasia. Because the researchers (who, collectively, spoke his three languages) lived in a different state from EC, long-distance treatment via the Internet was determined to be the most feasible solution. He agreed to participate in the study when the possibility of employing the Internet to conduct the study long-distance was proposed to him.

Assessment. Multiple baseline measurements were collected, allowing us to measure EC's morphosyntax and language production rate before and after each treatment block. We consider these multiple baselines because (a) we repeatedly measured treated and non-treated skills (morphosyntax and speech rate) prior to and following each treatment block (which focused on morphosyntax and language production rate, respectively), and (b) because we collected measurements in the treated language, English (L2), and in the two non-treated languages, Hebrew (L1) and French (L3). The same measurements were collected three times on each of five occasions: before treatment began (Baseline), following the first treatment block (Post Treatment 1), before the second treatment block and after a period of no treatment (Pre Treatment 2), following the second treatment block (Post Treatment 2), and 6 months after the end of the second treatment block (Follow-up). At each point of data collection we obtained three measurements on two or three consecutive days to confirm performance stability, each comprising several tasks. For the purpose of the present paper we report data from an elicited sentence production task.

For the elicited sentence production task (used for assessment only), we employed a selection of 60 pictures from the Sentence Production Program for Aphasia (SPPA; Helm-Estrabrooks & Nicholas, 2000) (the SPPA had not been used for treatment with EC). We used the picture stimuli from the SPPA but not the target responses provided in the SPPA manual. Instead, EC was directed to one picture at a time and instructed to describe in two sentences what he saw happening in the picture. (For example, he was shown the picture of a man in a swimming pool and a woman sitting at the edge of that pool. The clinician instructed him to describe in two sentences what was going on in the picture. EC said: "The man in the pool eh tell his wife: come in the pool and swim with me. The woman says: it's too cold for me"). Different subsets of 12 pictures were used in an alternating fashion for the three languages during the differing measurement points, yielding 24 sentences per administration in each language (for examples, see Appendix). Over the course of testing, the same picture stimuli were presented in the three languages.

Because EC's language skills were only mildly impaired, and because treatment targeted sentence production in discourse context, we chose to assess his language skills before and after treatment with this rather open-ended task. In contrast to the standard administration of the SPPA, our aim was to examine EC's spontaneous sentence generation skills, rather than his ability to produce pre-determined sentence structures. The sentences EC generated were recorded and transcribed verbatim for analysis. The sentence production task allowed us to measure two aspects of EC's language production abilities: morphosyntactic accuracy and speech rate.

Analysis

Using the sentence elicited in each language we conducted the following two analyses. For each analysis, values for each sentence were obtained and means across the three measurements per occasion and across the five testing occasions were calculated.

Morphosyntactic coding. For this analysis each sentence produced by the participant in the sentence elicitation task was coded as "correct", "self-corrected", or "incorrect" on the following six morphosyntactic measures: Noun–Verb

Agreement, Tense Consistency, Prepositions, Pronoun–Gender Agreement, Sentence Complexity, and Overall Accuracy. For French sentences, Noun–Article Agreement was also examined. The number of possible occurrences for each measurement ranged from 2 to over 44, with over 90% of all measures having a minimum of 10 possible occurrences.

- Noun–Verb Agreement: Because the only English verb conjugation that requires overt morphological marking is the third person singular in the present tense, only those cases were counted as an opportunity for agreement. We tallied the percentage of correctly marked verb agreement (e.g., "The man ask*s* his wife ..."); that is, we calculated the number of instances of correct marking out of the number of opportunities to do so, multiplied by 100. For Hebrew and French sentences, possible occurrences included all persons and tenses because these languages mark verb agreement for different persons/genders.
- Tense Consistency: The percentage of times in which the participant maintained tense consistency across the two sentences he produced to describe a picture (e.g., "The man told his wife about the snow. He ask*ed* her ...") was examined.
- Prepositions: We tallied the percentage of correctly used prepositions out of all prepositions used (e.g., "The man asked: 'What is *in* the box?'").
- Pronoun–Gender Agreement: The percentage of correctly agreed pronouns was obtained for each sentence (e.g., "The man asked *his* wife.").
- Sentence complexity: We counted the proportions of complex versus simple sentences used across the total (24) sentences.
- Noun–Article Agreement: For the French production only, the percentage of correct agreement between the article and the noun following it (e.g., "*la* fille a dit ...") was examined.
- Overall Accuracy: Each sentence was marked as "correct", "self-correct", or "incorrect", taking into account the measures above plus word choice and other errors not included in the measures detailed above.

Speech rate (syllable-per-minute measurements). This analysis allowed us to assess the participant's overall language production rate. Because his language production was largely accurate but extremely slow, characterised by frequent hesitations, false starts, and self-corrections, we were interested in examining the effect of language treatment on his production rate. Therefore, for this analysis the duration of each sentence produced in the sentence elicitation task was measured. Sound Forge (Sony) software was employed to compute the duration of EC's sentences. Numbers were rounded to the nearest millisecond. Onset of speech (i.e., the beginning of a sentence or the end of a pause) was defined as a change in amplitude at the zero crossing of the waveform indicating the beginning of an utterance, whereas offset of speech (i.e., the end of a sentence or the beginning of a pause) was defined as a decrease in amplitude in the waveform corresponding to the end of an utterance, reaching the zero crossing. For each sentence we divided the duration in seconds by the number of syllables produced in the sentence to yield a syllable-per-minute measure. For the syllable count we included only the meaningful portion of the sentence, excluding false starts, repetitions, and fillers.

For each of the analyses, a trained research assistant who was a native speaker or a highly proficient speaker of the analysed language completed the data coding for all measurements. A second trained individual completed the coding for 2 (13%) of the 15 (three per each of five occasions) measurements. Inter-rater reliability for the transcriptions, morphosyntactic coding, sentence duration, and syllable count ranged from 85% to 99%.

Following the analyses we tabulated the values obtained per measurement and the means of the three repeated measurements per testing occasion. To assess change, we calculated the effect size (Beeson & Robey, 2006) of the difference between occasions. For example, to assess change following the first treatment block we subtracted the average of Baseline (Pre-treatment 1) from the average of Post-treatment 1 and divided the difference by the standard deviation of Baseline. Differences between two occasions that yielded an effect size greater than 1 are taken as substantial and reported here.[2]

RESULTS

Results will be described first for English (L2), the treated language, and then for Hebrew (L1) and French (L3).

English (L2), the treated language

Morphosyntactic coding. Following the first treatment block (morphosyntax), the accuracy of Noun–Verb Agreement increased from 57% to 73% (effect size=1.6), and of Pronoun Gender Agreement from 91% to 100% (effect size=1.8) (see Figure 2). In addition, the percentage of Overall Accuracy increased from 32% to 44% (effect size=1.2). The accuracy percentage of correct Tense Consistency, Prepositions, and the percentage of Complex Sentences used did not change.

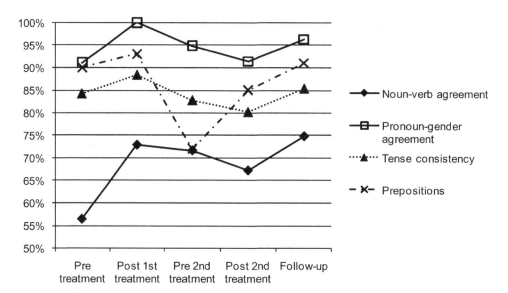

Figure 2. Percent accuracy of morphosyntactic structures in English (L2, the treated language).

---

[2] Previous studies of aphasia treatment in a single-participant design report larger effect sizes for trained items tested before and after treatment than the ones we found here. We assessed change using untrained items in a free sentence elicitation task and therefore would expect small effect sizes.

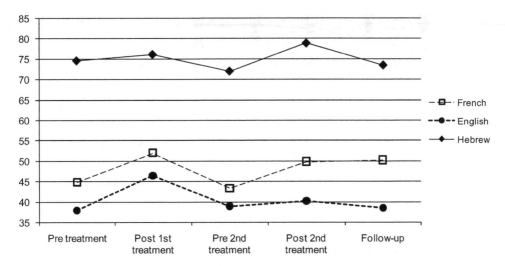

Figure 3. Number of syllables per minute (on the Y axis) in the treated language and the two non-treated languages.

Following the second treatment block (language production rate), the only change noted was an increase in the percentage accurate Preposition use from 72% to 85% (effect size=1.7). No other measures showed change following the second treatment block.

Speech rate. The number of syllables per minute (per sentence) increased from 37.84 to 46.36 (effect size=1.2), following the first treatment block (morphosyntax) (see Figure 3). There was no change following the second treatment block (language production rate) (from 38.86 to 40.15) (effect size <1).

The non-treated languages: Hebrew (L1)

Morphosyntactic coding. EC demonstrated high accuracy levels (ranging from 91% to 100%) on the measures analysed, with no marked change across measurements (see Figure 4).

Speech rate. There was no significant change in the number of syllables per minute in Hebrew following the first or the second treatment blocks (from 74.41 to 75.99 and from 78.76 to 73.29, respectively) (see Figure 3).

The non-treated languages: French (L3)

Morphosyntactic coding. Following the first treatment block (morphosyntax), there was an increase in the accuracy rates in French for Prepositions from 78% to 95% (effect size=1.4); for Pronoun–Gender Agreement from 74% to 88% (effect size=2.1); and Tense Consistency from 68% to 83% (effect size=1.9) (see Figure 5). Overall Accuracy increased from 32% to 49% (effect size=2.9).

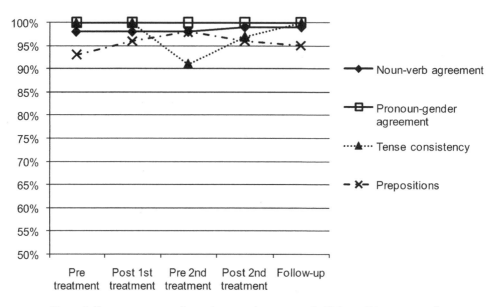

Figure 4. Percent accuracy of morphosyntactic structures in Hebrew (L1, non-treated).

Following the second treatment block (language production rate), the only measures that showed change were Tense Consistency from 72% to 94% (effect size=2.8), and Overall accuracy from 26% to 49% (effect size=2.6).

Speech rate. As in English, the number of syllables per minute increased in French following the first treatment block (morphosyntax) (see Figure 3). The increase was from 44.77 to 51.86 (effect size=1.6). No significant change was noted following the second treatment block (language production rate) (from 43.31 to 49.77) (effect size <1).

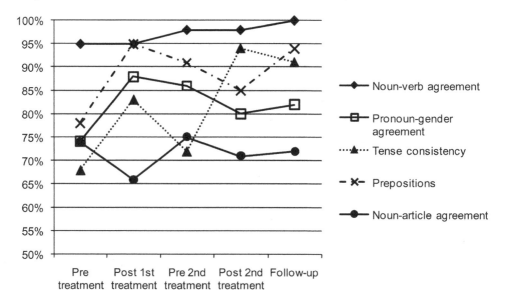

Figure 5. Percent accuracy of morphosyntactic structures in French (L3, non-treated).

DISCUSSION

In this study we contrasted two blocks of language treatment administered to a trilingual speaker with chronic nonfluent aphasia to examine how language status (cross-language generalisation to L1 vs to L3) and the language aspects being treated (morphosyntactic vs language production rate) influence cross-language treatment generalisation. The treatment was administered in English, the participant's second language. We collected pre-and post-treatment measurements in the treated language as well as in the two non-treated languages: the participant's first language, Hebrew, and his third language, French. The results demonstrated that in response to the first treatment block (morphosyntax), there was a small increase in accuracy rates for selected morphosyntactic components in English, the treated language. A small increase in English speech rate following the first treatment block was also found. These findings suggest that a treatment approach that emphasises informative exchanges between the client and the clinician yields positive outcomes in individuals with chronic aphasia. Furthermore, the treatments employed were, in part, metalinguistic in nature (e.g., explicitly addressing morphosyntactic rules), in accordance with the participant's mild impairment and his good metalinguistic skills.

Additionally, as in English, the treated language, increased morphosyntactic accuracy and speech rate following the first treatment block (morphosynatx) were found also in French, the participant's non-treated third language. These increases following the treatment block that focused on morphosyntactic skills in English are suggestive of cross-language treatment generalisation from L2 to L3. Two portions of the findings corroborate our assumption that the improvement in French can be attributed to the treatment in English. One is the fact that the increase in accuracy rates in Prepositions, Pronoun–Gender Agreement, and Tense Consistency in French were found following the first treatment period, the treatment that focused on such morphosyntactic elements, and were generally not found following the second treatment block in which the focus was on language production rate. The second is the finding that no improvement was found in the French rates of Article–Noun agreement,[3] a morphosyntactic component that does not exist in English. This latter finding suggests that cross-language generalisation is more likely for language components that exist in both the treated and the non-treated languages than for components that differ in the two languages.

We note that the increase in English and French speech rate followed the first treatment block (morphosynatx) but not the second (language production rate). This suggests to us that, in part, the participant's speech rate is slowed by his struggle with morphosyntactic language components. Therefore treating morphosyntactic skills in individuals with non-fluent aphasia may not only enhance their grammatical production but also their production rate. In this case we argue that a treatment approach that targets specific language components can yield an improvement in functional communication. We acknowledge that the magnitude of change observed following treatment was small. We might have expected small effect sizes in our data because we measured the participant's performance on untrained items in a relatively

---

[3] We note that, on average, 60% of the nouns analysed for the Article–Noun agreement in French were animate nouns and about 50% of EC's Article–Noun agreement errors were on animate nouns. Most nouns (mean 97%) were singular nouns.

open-ended task (compared to effect sizes obtained for trained items in a picture naming test, see, for example, Wright, Marshall, Wilson, & Page, 2007).

We did not find a significant increase in Hebrew morphosyntactic accuracy or speech rates following either treatment block. This finding can be explained by at least two factors. One is the high performance rate in Hebrew, the participant's first and most recovered language. That is, we can assume that cross-language generalisation was not found due to ceiling performance in Hebrew. This is true for the morphosyntactic measures we used. In contrast, the participant's speech rate in Hebrew (around 80 syllables per minute) is still well below typical speech rate (120–200 words per minute). Alternatively, it could be hypothesised that due to the status of Hebrew as the participant's first language, there was differential representation and processing of Hebrew and English, and therefore there was no cross-language generalisation between these two languages. Unlike for Hebrew, cross-language generalisation was found between English and French, the two languages that were non-L1. Certainly, English and French may be expected to have more shared structures and representations at the lexical level than English and Hebrew, due to shared origins. Yet the role of structural and lexical similarities in cross-language treatment generalisation is still largely undetermined. For example, lexical similarities were deemed to be critical in determining cross-language generalisation in Kohnert's (2004) study, whereas cross-language generalisation has also been documented for languages that share few structural and lexical elements (e.g., English and Japanese in Watamori & Sasanuma, 1978).

With respect to our predictions, we found that the participant showed treatment-related gains in the skills addressed in the treated language (L2). In addition, in contrast to the prediction that overlapping representation and processing of languages of high proficiency would lead to cross-language generalisation to both the participant's L1 and L3, we found treatment-related improvement only in French, the participant's L3, and not in L1, Hebrew. Rather, the prediction that language status affects the occurrence of cross-language treatment generalisation was supported by the data. That is, we found a differential pattern of cross-language generalisation for the non-treated L1 vs the non-treated L3. This difference in language status is confounded by a difference in degree of recovery of the two non-treated languages, as well as the structural relations between each language pair. Furthermore, the participant's near-ceiling performance on the Hebrew morpho-syntactic structures precludes an unequivocal conclusion regarding cross-language generalisation to the participant's L1 (similar results are reported for L1 in Miertsch, Meisel, & Isel, 2009). To dissociate these factors, additional studies with bilingual and multilingual speakers of other sets of languages are warranted in which, for example, the two non-treated languages would be equally impaired or equally related to the treated language.

Our findings of cross-language generalisation from the participant's more-recovered language to a less-recovered language can be taken as inconsistent with Edmonds and Kiran's (2006) findings. However, their study focused on lexical retrieval abilities, whereas our cross-language findings concerned morphosyntactic skills.

Our study has several limitations. Because of the near-ceiling performance on our morphosyntactic measures in Hebrew, and because of the differences in structural similarities among the three languages, it is difficult to ascertain the reason for the differential cross-language generalisation found for French and Hebrew. Furthermore, because we did not find improvement in the treated language following the second treatment block (language production rate), we were unable to fully contrast cross-language effects of the two treatment blocks. The small improvement we measured following treatment can be attributed to the assessment task we used (a sentence elicitation task, measuring performance on newly elicited sentences rather than trained items) and to a relatively short treatment period. Further study will be useful to answer these unresolved questions.

CONCLUSION

The data from this within-participant treatment study suggest a complex pattern of generalisation from the treated language to the non-treated languages of a trilingual speaker with mild chronic aphasia. Change in the speaker's morphosyntactic performance was noted in the treated language (English, L2), as well as in certain aspects of his production in the non-treated French, his third language. Clinically, the results of this study suggest that treating individuals in one of their languages (at least when emphasising informative exchanges and addressing metalinguistic aspects of language production) could benefit their non-treated language. The investigation of treatment effects in bilingual and multilingual individuals represents a fertile area of clinical research, which could help determine the efficacy of treating individuals with aphasia in their non-native language.

REFERENCES

Abutalebi, J., Cappa, S., & Perani, D. (2001). The bilingual brain as revealed by functional neuroimaging. *Bilingualism: Language and Cognition, 4*, 179–190.

Abutalebi, J., & Green, D. (2007). Bilingual language production: The neurocognition of language representation and control. *Journal of Neurolinguistics, 20*, 242–275.

Beeson, P. M., & Robey, R. (2006). Evaluating single-subject treatment research: Lessons learned from the aphasia literature. *Neuropsychological Review, 16*, 161–169.

Chee, M. W. L., Tan, E. W. L., & Thiel, T. (1999). Mandarin and English single word processing studied with functional magnetic resonance imaging. *Journal of Neuroscience, 19*, 3050–3056.

Diaz, C. J. (2003). Latino/a voices in Australia: Negotiating bilingual identity. *Contemporary Issues in Early Childhood, 4*, 314–336.

Edmonds, L., & Kiran, S. (2006). Effects of semantic naming treatment on crosslinguistic generalisation in bilingual aphasia. *Journal of Speech Language and Hearing Research, 49*, 729–748.

Friederici, A. D. (2004). The neural basis of syntactic processes. In M. Gazzaniga (Ed.), *The cognitive neurosciences III* (pp. 803–814). Cambridge, MA: MIT Press.

Friederici, A. D., Hahne, A., & von Cramon, D. Y. (1998). First-pass versus second-pass parsing processes in a Wernicke's and a Broca's aphasic: Electrophysiological evidence for a double dissociation. *Brain and Language, 62*, 311–341.

Gil, M., & Goral, M. (2004). Non-parallel recovery in bilingual aphasia: Effects of language choice, language proficiency, and treatment. *International Journal of Bilingualism, 8*, 191–219.

Goral, M., & Kempler, D. (in press). Training verb production in communicative context: Evidence from a person with chronic non-fluent aphasia. *Aphasiology*.

Goral, M., Levy, E. S., Obler, L. K., & Cohen, E. (2006). Lexical connections in the multilingual lexicon. *Brain and Language, 98*, 235–247.

Helm-Estabrooks, N., & Nicholas, M. (2000). *Sentence Production Program for Aphasia*. Austin, TX: Pro-Ed.

Jochmann, A. (2006). Speech and language treatment in East Africa. *The ASHA Leader, 11*(2), 8–9, 32–33.

Kohnert, K. (2004). Cognitive and cognate-based treatments for bilingual aphasia: A case study. *Brain and Language, 91*, 294–302.

Lalor, E., & Kirsner, K. (2001). The role of cognates in bilingual aphasia: Implications for assessment and treatment. *Aphasiology, 15*, 1047–1056.

Levy, E. S., Crowley, C. J., Wagner, E. M., Downey, S., Kastl, R., & Pleshivoy, Y. et al. (2007). *SLP students with accents: University clinics' policies and practices.* Poster presented at the American Speech-Language-Hearing Convention, Boston, MA.

Meinzer, M., Elbert, T., Djundja, D., Taub, E., & Rockstroh, B. (2007). Extending the Constraint-Induced Movement Therapy (CIMT) approach to cognitive functions: Constraint-Induced Aphasia Therapy (CIAT) of chronic aphasia. *NeuroRehabilitation, 22*, 311–318.

Mennen, I., & Stansfield, J. (2006). Speech and language therapy service delivery for bilingual children: A survey of three cities in Great Britain. *International Journal of Language and Communication Disorders, 41*, 635–652.

Miertsch, B., Meisel, J., & Isel, F. (2009). Non-treated languages is aphasia therapy of polyglots benefit from improvement in the treated language. *Journal of Neurolinguistics, 22*(2), 135–150.

Paradis, M. (1983). *Reading on aphasia in polyglots.* Montreal: Didier.

Paradis, M. (1993). Bilingual aphasia rehabilitation. In M. Paradis (Ed.), *Foundations of aphasia rehabilitation.* Oxford, UK: Pergamon Press.

Paradis, M. (2004). *A neurolinguistic theory of bilingualism.* Amsterdam: John Benjamins Publishing Company.

Paradis, M., & Libben, G. (1987). *The assessment of bilingual aphasia.* Hillsdale, NJ: Lawrence Erlbaum Associates Inc.

Perani, D., & Abutalebi, J. (2005). Neural basis of first and second language processing. *Current Opinion of Neurobiology, 15*, 202–206.

Roberts, P. M. (2008). Aphasia assessment and treatment for bilingual and culturally diverse patients. In R. Chapey (Ed.), *Language intervention strategies for aphasia and related neurogenic communication disorders* (5th ed., pp. 245–276). New York: Lippincott, Williams & Wilkins.

Ullman, M. T. (2006). The declarative/procedural model and the shallow structure hypothesis. *Applied Psycholinguistics, 27*, 97–105.

Ullman, M. T., Pancheva, R., Love, T., Yee, E., Swinney, D., & Hickok, G. (2005). Neural correlates of lexicon and grammar: Evidence from the production, reading, and judgment of inflection in aphasia. *Brain and Language, 93*, 185–238.

Vaid, J., & Hull, H. (2002). Re-envisioning the bilingual brain using functional neuroimaging: Methodological and interpretive issues. In F. Fabbro (Ed.), *Advances in the neurolinguistics of bilingualism.* Udine, Italy: Forum.

Watamori, T. S., & Sasanuma, S. (1978). The recovery processes of two English–Japanese bilingual aphasics. *Brain and Language, 6*, 127–140.

Wiener, D., Obler, L. K., & Taylor-Sarno, M. (1995). Speech/language management of the bilingual aphasic in a U.S. urban rehabilitation hospital. In M. Paradis (Ed.), *Aspects of bilingual aphasia* (pp. 37–56). Tarrytown, NY: Elsevier.

Winter, K. (1999). Speech and language therapy provision for bilingual children: Aspects of the current service. *International Journal of Language and Communication Disorders, 34*, 85–98.

Wright, H. H., Marshall, R. C., Wilson, K. B., & Page, J. L. (2007). Using a written cueing hierarchy to improve verbal naming in aphasia. *Aphasiology, 22*, 522–536.

APPENDIX: Examples of EC's responses to the elicited sentence task

English (*Responses to 12 pictures (pre-treatment 1, first baseline measurement)*)

SPPA Picture 17:
Umm the old man ask his wife uhhh uhh can his wife to lie sofa. Uhhh uh the woman umm tell told her husband that she has a severe headache.

SPPA Picture 19:
Uhh the young player umm had a homerun uhhh homerun. Ummm the the woman umm ummm umm the side umm ummm eh shouted: Homerun!

SPPA Picture 21:
Don't uhhh uhh don't don't put in your mouth the corner. Ummm and the young woman tell her dog: Don't stay here in the apartment.

SPPA Picture 23:
Ummm the young woman umm tell tell told her friends about last night. Ehhh emmm she had a wonderful night with her new boyfriend.

SPPA Picture 25:
Umm Bill is uhh thinking about his trip. He doesn't look ehh to the wall uh ball.

SPPA Picture 47:
Uhhh umm the dad uhhh tell his son about the soup that he ummm makes. And ehh the young boy thinks the soup that his dad is making is uhhh ummm is beer.

SPPA Picture 49:
Uhhh the the young man fell from the ladder. He is confused.

SPPA Picture 51: Umm the old man uhh uhhh wants to drink red wine. He uhhh hates the ummm noodles that the his wife uhhh brings.

SPPA Picture 53:
The doctor ummm ehhh umm show shows the the young patient uhhh the thermometer. The young doctor said says that he she doesn't want the thermometer.

SPPA Picture 55:
Umm uhh play with me ummm umm poker. The old man uhh says to his wife: let's play.

SPPA Picture 77:
The father wants to know ehh whether the his sons uhhh played basketball. The the Alan says to his father: eh I we uhh played through the ball eh to the basket.

SPPA Picture 79:
The the young man ummm ask his father: what's what are you doing? I want you to uhh ummm work ehhh in my room.

Hebrew

17:

אה אה ה איש הזקן אה מראה ל אישה שלו את הספה. אה הוא אומר לה אה תש אה תשכבי על הספה.

:19

האיש אה הנער מרוצה מה אה מכה שהוא נתן ל כדור בייסבול שלו אה ה כדור הבייסבול.

אה הוא אה אמר אה הוא צועק: אה אה "הומראן".

:21

הנערה אומרת לכלב: תישאר פה בבית. אני אה צריכה לצאת עם החבר שלי.

:23

ה ילדה מספרת על על הח על ה לחברה שלה אה אה אה מה היה ה ביום ש שעבר אה ב בין אה סיגל אה לחבר

שלה. ה ה החברה שלה אומרת: תשתקי.

:25

ה ילד ה אה אה הילד שיש לו שריון על החזה אומר לילד ל חבר שלו אה אה אה תפסיק עם ה אה תפסיק עם ה

חשיבה ה תיאורטית אה שלך. אה יש אה מתקרב לפה כדור.

:47

אה ה אבא אומר ל ילד שלו אה תביא לי מים. אה צריך להוסיף מים ל מרק.

:49

ה אמא אומרת ל ילד: תצלצל אפס אחד אחד אה תשע אחד אחד. אה תבקש אה תגיד להם ש אבא נפל.

:51

ה א הבעל שואל את האישה שלו אה למה צריך צריך אה אה אה צריך ה הלמה צריך שה מפה תהיה ה לוח השח

שלי? אה האישה אומרת אה אה אה אה תפסיק לדבר שטויות.

:53

ה איש אה ה דוקטור אה מוציא את ה מודד חום ונותן ל נערה. אה הנערה אומרת: איכס

:55

האישה שואלת את הבעל שלה: אה אה אפשר לשחק איתך בקלפים? ה בעל שלה אומר: איזה משחקקלף..

קלפים?

:77

האבא אומר: אה אני רוצה לשחק איתכם כדורסל. מה החוקים של משחקהכדורסל?

:79

ה האיש הזקן אומר לבן שלו יש לי אה אה אה תביא לי קרשים. אה אני אה חסר ליקרשרים קרשים אה אה ל גג של

הבית ש ה הזה שאני בונה.

French

<u>17</u> :
Euh la femme a dit à son mari euh tu as euh euh euh euh tu as la tête en bas et le et la jambe en haut. Et euh la le mari a dit pourquoi?

<u>19</u> :
La le l'entraîneur l'entraîneuse a dit à son euh à son euh à sa euh membre de l'équipe euh euh bravo. euh alain (?) euh tu as euh famé (?)

<u>21</u> :
La le chien a a dit à sa euh au a à la femme euh est ce que je peux euh manger le fruit ?
Euh la femme a dit à son chien euh euh euh ces fruits euh ils sont euh euh c'est une peinture euh pas le vrai fruit.

<u>23</u> :
Euh le la jeune femme a euh ra euh raconté à sa son amie euh euh euh le de euh euh de .... le la fête euh de de hier. Euh euh la le la copine a dit euh euh stp euh euh euh je euh euh euh veux euh que tu euh ra raconte moi encore euh euh euh stp euh donne un euh un .... Partons euh tout de suite un dehors dehors pour euh pour me raconter la suite.

<u>25</u> :
Euh euh la le le garçon qui euh a le euh armoire (?) ? .... euh le machin qui euh sur le la ventre euh a dit à son copain euh tu euh rêves. Euh le il y a une balle qui vient euh euh vers toi.

<u>47</u> :
Euh euh la le père la le papa a dit à son fils, euh euh moi j'ai fait euh la soupe à deux personnes. Euh euh la fils a dit non papa.

<u>49</u> :
Euh la femme a dit à son mari euh quel combien de euh euh arbres il y a? Euh euh le mari a dit il y a euh un arbre euh ombre.

<u>51</u> :
Euh la le mari euh le la femme a dit à son mari c'est ton anniversaire. Euh euh euh j'ai euh cuisiné euh les nouilles.

<u>53</u> :
La le médecin a dit à sa euh à une euh à la fille euh euh c'est une sucette. Euh euh euh mets ça euh dans dans ta bouche.

<u>55</u>:
La femme a dit à sa à son mari: où est euh le chat. Euh le la le mari à dit euh le chat est sur mes ... jambes.

<u>77</u> :
Le la père est dans ... la père a dit à ses fils euh euh euh quel est le score?
Euh un fils a dit à son père euh c'est 0-0.

<u>79</u> :
Euh la fils a dit à son papa quel euh modèle tu construis? Euh la le papa a dit à son fils euh euh ce modèle est euh euh est ta euh maison.

APHASIOLOGY, 2010, 24 (2), 210–230

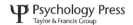

Action and object naming versus verb and noun retrieval in connected speech: Comparisons in late bilingual Greek–English anomic speakers

Maria Kambanaros

Technological Educational Institute of Patras, Greece

Background: Recently, verb–noun processing differences were reported in a group of late bilingual speakers with fluent, anomic aphasia in Greek (L1) as well as in English (L2) (Kambanaros & van Steenbrugge, 2006). The findings revealed that verb production was significantly more impaired than noun production in both languages during picture naming despite preserved comprehension of action and object names.
Aims: The aim of this study is to investigate the total number (quantity) and the diversity (quality or different types) of verbs and nouns produced in conversational speech by the same group of bilingual anomic individuals with aphasia and compare the results to (i) those of the non-brain-injured control group and (ii) their action and object naming performances at the single word level, to determine if grammatical class impairments are also evident in spontaneous speech.
Methods & Procedures: In order to examine the distribution and diversity of verbs and nouns in spontaneous speech, speech samples of 300 words were collected from the bilingual individuals with fluent aphasia and their controls in L1 and in L2 on two separate occasions, 1 week apart. In addition, two subtests from the Greek Object and Action Test (GOAT: Kambanaros, 2003), the object and action naming subtests, were presented on two separate occasions, 1 week apart, to both groups of bilingual participants in L1 and L2 (cf. Kambanaros & van Steenbrugge, 2006).
Outcomes & Results: Late bilingual participants with anomia showed no difficulties retrieving verbs in spontaneous speech in L1 or L2 despite a significant verb deficit in both languages on action naming tasks. However the bilingual group had significant difficulties in relation to noun production in spontaneous speech in L1 and L2.
Conclusions: Picture naming remains the standard of word retrieval ability in aphasia. However, object and action naming scores can underestimate and/or overestimate word retrieval performance for nouns and verbs in connected speech.

Keywords: Naming; Spontaneous speech; Bilingual aphasia.

The aim of this study is to investigate verb and noun production in conversational speech and compare it to confrontation naming performance in a group of late bilingual individuals with anomic aphasia who speak Greek (L1) and English (L2). Apart from the opportunity to investigate language-specific deficits regarding verb and noun lexical retrieval, Greek–English bilingual aphasia is also interesting because of the linguistic differences between the two languages. Like English, Greek

Address correspondence to: Maria Kambanaros PhD, Department of Speech and Language Therapy, School of Health and Welfare, Technological Educational Institute of Patras, Megalou Alexandrou 1, Koukouli 26334 Patras, Greece. E-mail: kambanarou@teipat.gr is a stem-based language but with a more complex morphology. Unlike English, stems in Greek serve as representational units rather than actual words. For example, the Greek stem *"kov–"* of the verb *"kovo"* (translation *I cut*) carries some semantic features but no meaning, as the stem does not have inflection, whereas the stem of a verb in English (e.g. *cut*) does have meaning. Therefore word meanings and grammatical category are derived from the suffix in Greek; that is, lexical class words (e.g., nouns, verbs) receive syntactic and semantic information following inflection.

For close to four decades, researchers have continued to investigate verb–noun word retrieval distinctions in monolingual speakers. Their findings reinforce earlier claims that selective verb impairments are mainly found in nonfluent, agrammatic patients with an anterior cortical lesion that includes Broca's area (Berndt, Haendiges, Mitchum & Sandson, 1997a; Breedin et al., 1998; Breen & Warrington, 1994; Kim & Thompson, 2000; Manning & Warrington, 1996; McCarthy & Warrington, 1985; Marshall, Pring, & Chiat, 1998; Shapiro, Shelton, & Caramazza, 2000; Zingeser & Berndt, 1990). This holds true for languages other than English such as Chinese (Bates, Chen, Tzeng, Li, & Opie, 1991), Danish (Jensen, 2000), Dutch (Bastiaanse, 1991; Jonkers, 1998; Jonkers & Bastiaanse, 1996), Finnish (Laine, Kujala, Niemi, & Uusipaikka, 1992), German (De Bleser & Kauschke, 2002), Hungarian (Osman-Sagi, 1987), Italian (Daniele, Guistolisi, Silveri, Colosimo, & Gainotti, 1994; Luzzati et al., 2002; Miceli, Silveri, Noncentini, & Caramazza, 1988; Miceli, Silveri, Villa, & Caramazza, 1984; Silveri & Di Betta, 1997) and Greek (Tsapkini, Jarema, & Kehayia, 2002).

Researchers have also found the opposite pattern for patients with posterior lesions of the left hemisphere; that is, impaired noun retrieval with relatively spared verb naming. Again this has been demonstrated for a number of languages: English (Berndt et al., 1997a; Berndt, Haendiges, & Wozniak, 1997b; Breen & Warrington, 1994; Caramazza & Hillis, 1991; Shapiro et al., 2000; Zingeser & Berndt, 1990), Chinese (Bates et al., 1991; Chen & Bates, 1998), French (Bachoud-Levi & Dupoux, 2003), Italian (Daniele et al., 1994; Luzzatti et al., 2002; Miceli et al., 1984; Miozzo, Soardi, & Cappa, 1994), and Hungarian (Osman-Sagi, 1987). In addition there are reports of selective verb deficits in participants who have fluent aphasia in languages such as: Dutch (Bastiaanse & Jonkers, 1998; Jonkers, 1998; Jonkers & Bastiaanse, 1996), English (Berndt & Haendiges, 2000; Berndt et al., 1997a; McCann & Edwards, 2002), German (De Bleser & Kauschke, 2002), Italian (Luzzatti et al., 2002), and Greek (Kambanaros, 2007; Tsapkini et al., 2002).

Contrary to the above findings, a number of other studies have demonstrated greater difficulty with verb processing compared to noun processing regardless of lesion site (anterior or posterior). This is reported in English (Berndt et al., 1997a; Caramazza & Hillis, 1991; Daniele et al., 1994; Hillis & Caramazza, 1995; Kohn, Lorch, & Pearson, 1989; Manning & Warrington, 1996; Marshall et al., 1998; McCarthy & Warrington, 1985; Williams & Canter, 1987), Dutch (Bastiaanse & Jonkers, 1998; Jonkers & Bastiaanse, 1996), French (Kremin, 1994), and Italian (Basso, Razzano, Faglioni, & Zanobio, 1990).

Despite the plethora of studies, little is known about the retrieval of different types of verbs and nouns or the factors influencing their retrieval, even after many years of research. Many factors have led to the contradictory outcomes and include the findings that: (i) verbs and nouns are highly variable in meaning but can also have a close relationship (e.g., instrumentality, name relation); (ii) lesion studies linking verb–noun dissociations to specific brain areas are controversial; (iii) methodological issues including participant selection criteria and test construction are not always reported or controlled for; and (iv) verb–noun differences have been studied in languages with different underlying forms. In spite of the complexity and contradictions, the finding that grammatical class effects may arise in participants with aphasia is robust. According to Luzzatti and colleagues (2002, p. 442):

> ... verb-noun dissociations cannot be simply discarded as an artifact resulting from unbalanced word frequency or imageability, but have to be accepted as a genuine part-of-speech effect.

Some researchers have noted different patterns of verbs and noun retrieval depending on the retrieval context; that is, retrieval in *single word* versus *sentences* and/or *connected speech*. For example, Manning and Warrington (1996) described a participant who was able to name objects in a picture-naming task but was unable to name the same objects in a sentence completion task. The reverse has also been reported; that is, a participant who was poor at naming single objects showed improved object naming when he was asked to produce object names using a sentence completion task (Zingeser & Berndt, 1988). In contrast, Jonkers and Bastiaanse (1998) described two fluent participants with a selective verb disorder at the single word level but no such deficit in connected speech.

Among the first studies to report differences in word retrieval for individuals with aphasia, in naming and connected speech contexts, were those conducted by Williams and Canter in studies going back 25 years involving monolingual English speakers with aphasia. In their first study (Williams & Canter, 1982), they reported the lowest association between object (noun) naming and noun retrieval in connected speech ($r = .54$) in a group of anomic individuals compared to other groups (Broca's, Wernicke's, and conduction aphasia). A similar finding was reported in a follow up study 5 years later (Williams & Canter, 1987) investigating verb retrieval: the anomic group had the lowest correlation for verb naming and verb retrieval in spontaneous speech ($r = .55$). Both results revealed that noun and verb retrieval in naming and in spontaneous speech were affected by retrieval context. Furthermore, the authors suggest that aphasia type may serve as a clinical marker in determining the relationship between confrontation naming and word retrieval in spontaneous speech.

Additional studies conducted on monolingual English speakers with anomia who present with a grammatical word class deficit for nouns in naming tasks reported better lexical retrieval performance in connected speech when compared to naming (Berndt et al., 1997a; Breen & Warrington, 1994; Zingeser & Berndt, 1990) and/or fewer word-finding difficulties for both nouns and verbs in connected speech than in naming (Mayer & Murray, 2003; Pashek & Tompkins, 2002; Williams & Canter, 1987). However, the opposite has been reported; that is, significantly worse word retrieval performance in conversation when compared to confrontation naming (Manning & Warrington, 1996).

The relationship between confrontation naming for verbs and/or nouns versus retrieval in connected speech has been investigated in languages other than English. Bastiaanse and Jonkers (1998) reported no significant correlations between verb retrieval in a naming test versus spontaneous speech in a group of monolingual Dutch individuals with anomia. A similar finding was reported by Basso et al. (1990)

for monolingual speakers of Italian with both verbs and nouns.[1] Luzzatti, Ingignoli, Crepaldi, and Semenza (2006) reported findings for noun and verb picture naming and noun/verb retrieval in spontaneous production for monolingual speakers of Italian with fluent aphasia. Differential patterns of performance were identified for each group and a difference between contexts for the verb-impaired individuals. The three noun-impaired fluent participants showed impaired noun retrieval on both the naming task and in spontaneous production, whereas the two verb-impaired individuals retrieved a normal amount of verbs in spontaneous speech despite poor performances on the verb picture naming task.

Relatively little is known about how bilingual individuals with aphasia process verbs and nouns. However, there is a wealth of information available on language recovery and localisation of both languages and on differential performance(s) in the two languages. Bilingual aphasia is of interest because one can test whether findings are an artefact of the specific language or have a wider application, namely that they apply to both languages. Five studies have been found in the literature investigating verb and noun differences in bilingual patients: three studies involve patients with a fluent and/or anomic aphasia resulting from left hemisphere lesions, one study reports noun–verb dissociations in an individual with Alzheimer's disease, and the other reports grammatical class differences following onset of primary progressive aphasia. A summary of studies describing grammatical word class effects in language-impaired bilingual adults is presented in Table 1.

In the first study a single case of a trilingual participant with word-finding difficulties in all three languages was reported. However, verb and noun retrieval were probed using picture naming only in the participant's second language, Italian. Both action and object words were retrieved equally well (97% and 93% respectively) thus not revealing a grammatical class effect as observed with monolingual patients. The researchers claimed that their finding substantiated two earlier assumptions from the monolingual literature: that action naming is not necessarily significantly preserved in anomia (Basso et al., 1990) and that there is no direct relationship between selective verb–noun impairments and aphasia type (Kremin & Basso, 1993). However, this study is somewhat flawed. First, conclusions are based on the results of one participant who was assessed in only one of her three languages, Italian. The participant lived in Italy yet used all three languages prior to her illness for different purposes (employment, with family etc.) on a daily basis. Therefore results from one language only are not representative of the participant's verb–noun processing abilities in the other languages, especially in this case where the participant's linguistic abilities differed across her three languages after her illness. Her first language, Bergamasc, was better preserved than Italian, and her third language, German, was the most impaired. Second, the participant was not a "typical" individual with aphasia since her lesion in the left hemisphere was of unknown aetiology and not related to stroke or neurological impairment. She presented with anomia after many years of epilepsy followed by removal of a tumour from the right temporal lobe. Third, the assessment materials were based on action and object pictures originally constructed in French, a language with a different deep structure from Italian. Finally, the researchers controlled only for frequency (high frequency) of the test items. It is possible then that the participant's high action and object

---

[1] Basso et al. (1990) did not statistically analyse noun/verb retrieval differences within fluent and non-fluent subgroups. It is therefore difficult to extrapolate the exact findings for the fluent aphasic group.

TABLE 1

A summary of studies describing grammatical word class effects in language-impaired bilingual adults

Study	Gender	Diagnosis	Languages	Age of acquisition	Proficiency	Effects	Methodology
Kremin & De Agostini (1995)	1 female	Lesion in the left hemisphere of unknown aetiology	Bergamac (L1) Italian (L2) German (L3)	Early	High	Nouns=Verbs tested in L2 only	Picture naming
Sasanuma & Park (1995)	1 male	Left CVA	Korean (L1) Japanese (L2)	Early	High	Nouns=Verbs	Picture naming and spontaneous speech
Kambanaros & van Steenbrugge (2006)	8 males 4 females	Anomic aphasia (Left CVAs)	Greek (L1) English (L2)	Late	High	Nouns>Verbs	Picture naming
Hernandez et al. (2006)	1 female	Anomic (BDAE-Cookie theft picture) Alzheimer's disease	Catalan (L1) Spanish (L2)	Early	High	Nouns<Verbs	Picture naming
Hernandez et al. (2008)	1 male	Non-fluent agrammatic (BDAE-Cookie theft picture)Primary Progressive Aphasia	Spanish (L1) Catalan (L2)	Late	High	Nouns>Verbs	Picture naming: verbal and written

naming scores were the result of a frequency effect (i.e., words of high frequency were easier to retrieve).

Sasanuma and Park (1995) assessed naming in a fluent speaker with aphasia in two languages, Korean (L1) and Japanese (L2). They used an aphasia test in each language across four modalities (auditory, reading, oral production, and writing). They described greater word retrieval difficulties in L2 compared to L1 for verbs and nouns in picture naming and conversation. However the researchers failed to describe test items or results in each grammatical category (verbs/nouns) for either language. Therefore their results are more in tune with findings from language recovery studies rather than grammatical word class processing.

In the study by Kambanaros and van Steenbrugge (2006) potential selective noun and/or verb processing deficits were investigated in bilingual individuals with anomic aphasia, to determine whether or not any specific noun or verb impairments were confined to their first language (Greek) or could also be found in their second language (English). The findings revealed that verbs were more difficult to retrieve than nouns when naming pictures of actions and objects, irrespective of language used by bilingual speakers with aphasia. The results were not affected by overall (residual) language proficiency in the two languages, nor by word frequency and imageability. Kambanaros and van Steenbrugge suggest that verb impairment in both languages was a result of greater difficulty accessing the (morpho-)phonological representation (lexemes) of verbs. The similarity of verb impairment in the two languages as well as similarity in the types of naming errors suggested the same level of breakdown when producing words in either language. Although the naming deficit was more severe in the second language of the bilingual anomic speakers, findings could not be attributed to lower proficiency in L2. Overall, results suggested a genuine verb–noun dichotomy during single word production in bilingual individuals with anomic aphasia that was independent of overall, residual L1 and L2 proficiency.

Hernandez, Costa, Sebastian-Galles, Juncadella, and Rene (2006) reported a patient with Alzheimer's disease (AD) who presented worse performance in retrieving nouns compared to verbs on naming tasks in both Catalan (L1) and Spanish (L2) despite good comprehension for both word classes across languages. Similarly, Hernandez et al. (2008) reported a grammatical class deficit in a bilingual Spanish (L1)–Catalan (L2) patient with primary progressive aphasia (PPA) who presented with more difficulties in naming verbs than nouns in spoken and written naming tasks in both languages. Naming performance and error types for verbs were similar across both languages with a worse performance in L2. In these studies grammatical class deficits are seen in patients with different underlying brain pathology excluding stroke or a focal lesion. Both AD and PPA are progressive and degenerative diseases, the latter of unknown aetiology, that involve more extensive cerebral damage. It is therefore difficult to tease out deficits to semantic information (e.g., action and object knowledge) and impairments to lexical networks in the brain. Furthermore, grammatical class effects are reported in two languages (Spanish and Catalan) with similar morpho-syntactic complexity and phonological properties. This raises two points: (a) how word properties are stored and retrieved in typologically similar languages, and (b) the relationship between lexical and syntactic deficits in typologically similar languages. Given these questions, the aims of this study were:

1. to see if verb and/noun retrieval difficulties are present in spontaneous speech;
2. to compare the results from spontaneous speech with word naming scores for action and object names;
3. to determine if verb and/noun retrieval difficulties are language specific;
4. to determine whether any difficulties that arise are due to the morphological differences between the two languages;
5. to compare results with monolingual studies for cross-language similarities.

METHOD

Participants

A total of 12 Greek–English-speaking, late bilingual individuals (i.e., those who had acquired L2 in early adulthood upon migration to Australia) with fluent, anomic aphasia (8 males and 4 females, aged between 60 and 84 years) participated in this study. Individuals with aphasia were recruited from any one of the following places: major inner city hospitals, rehabilitation centres, (Greek) nursing homes, and government agencies, e.g., Ethnic Link. Overall, five individuals with aphasia were referred by speech pathologists while the remaining participants were recruited from hospital database systems by the author. Bilingual participants' inclusion criteria were as follows: aphasia for at least 3 months as a consequence of a single episode of a focal, unilateral lesion in the left hemisphere, adequate hearing and vision for test purposes, and being right-handed (by self-report). Participant exclusion criteria were as follows: history of neurological disease or brain injury, present and/or past mental illness including depression, history of alcohol/substance abuse, as well as hearing and/or visual impairments. Information regarding the participants with aphasia is presented in Appendix A. In addition, 12 participants without aphasia served as controls. No participant suffered from neurological, major visual, or auditory problems. All controls were right-handed. They were matched with individuals in the aphasia group on factors including age of English language acquisition, chronological age, gender, socio-economic status, and level of education. In addition, three control participants married to non-Greek wives were recruited to match participants with aphasia who were also married to non-Greek women. All control participants were right-handed. All participants were volunteers and had given written consent in accordance with Flinders Clinical Research Ethics Committee (FCREC), Flinders Medical Centre.

Assessment

All participants were assessed with the Boston Diagnostic Aphasia Examination BDAE (Goodglass & Kaplan, 1983) to determine the presence/absence of aphasia, and if aphasia was present to classify performance as non-fluent or fluent aphasia. The following subtests of the BDAE were used: (i) conversational and expository speech including describing the Cookie Theft picture and (ii) auditory comprehension and oral expression subtests (excluding reading subtests). The BDAE was administered in English and Greek (Goodglass & Kaplan, 1983; Tsolaki, 1997) to both groups of participants on two separate occasions. In most cases, bilingual participants with aphasia had not been diagnosed with the BDAE in English and no participant had been assessed in Greek. All control participants were administered the same subtests of the BDAE as the participants with aphasia in both languages, since at the time of testing no norms existed for Greek–English participants with aphasia: thus, results from controls were used as criteria for selection. All participants with aphasia were classified as (fluent) anomia in both languages. Mean performance on the BDAE for participants with aphasia and non-brain-injured individuals are displayed in Appendix B. All participants with aphasia had fluent aphasia that could be best characterised as anomia in both languages as confirmed by the author of this study, who is a speech-language pathologist. In addition two other measures, a case history and a self-rating scale, were used to confirm bilingual status of participating individuals. A comprehensive case history was collected from each individual ($N = 24$) by the author in the language of their choice. Information collected included demographic details, family history, language history, language use, and communication needs. Major emphasis was given to the section on language use that included specific questions related to with whom and in what situations bilingual participants spoke Greek and/or English.

All bilingual individuals had been living in Australia on average for 46 years (range 37–53 years). They had all acquired English as a second language at a later age, after puberty. No bilingual individual was educated in Australia, revealing that English was learnt informally; instead all had attended schooling in Greece. All bilingual participants used both Greek and English on a regular basis in their daily lives. Greek was predominantly used in the home with the spouse and immediate family (but not with grandchildren) and at cultural or religious events/settings. English was predominantly used in daily activities outside the home such as shopping, car/home maintenance, banking, medical/health issues etc. All participants considered themselves fluent speakers of English following their migration to Australia.

Language proficiency was also assessed indirectly by means of a self-report in response to a self-rating language scale (adapted from Weber-Fox & Neville, 1996). All participants were requested to rate their proficiency using a 5-point scale of poor, fair, good, very good, to excellent, in the following modalities: understanding; communicating/speaking; reading; writing. Case history and self-rating scales were necessary to determine whether participants with aphasia were fluent bilinguals pre-morbidly, i.e., whether they were speaking both languages on a regular basis. A family informant was asked to verify participants' language abilities for both languages prior to the stroke. The information from the self-rating scale is depicted in Table 2.

Materials

Two subtests from the Greek Object and Action Test (GOAT: Kambanaros, 2003), the object and action naming subtests, were presented. The subtests were previously piloted in a group of 20 non-brain-injured, bilingual Greek–English speakers aged between 55 and 75 years. Items named with 80% accuracy or more were included in the test. Both the noun and verb subtests contained 55 items each. Stimuli were concrete nouns and verbs depicted by photographs showing the object or the action. All items of the GOAT had a high imageability and familiarity as evidenced by the response accuracy in the pilot group of participants. Furthermore the stimulus items were controlled for instrumentality and name relation (see Kambanaros & van Steenbrugge, 2006). There were no significant differences between mean word

TABLE 2

Mean performance of bilingual participants with aphasia and non-brain-injured groups on the self-rating scale in Greek and English

	Language proficiency							
	Speaking		Understanding		Reading		Writing	
Participants	Greek	English	Greek	English	Greek	English	Greek	English
Aphasia								
Mean	3.5	2.6	4.0	2.8	3.3	1.5	2.7	1.3
Control								
Mean	5.0	4.6	5.0	4.8	4.6	3.4	4.5	3.4

BA = bilingual aphasic participant; BC = bilingual control participant; 1 = poor; 2 = average; 3 = good; 4 = very good; 5 = excellent.

frequencies for nouns (mean 89.31 per million) and verbs (mean 69.95 per million) across all subtests of the GOAT (Kucera & Francis, 1970). None of the Greek words in the test was an English cognate word.

Procedure

Spontaneous speech. In order to examine the distribution and diversity of verbs and nouns in spontaneous speech, speech samples of 300 words were collected from the individuals with bilingual fluent aphasia and their controls in L1 and in L2 on two separate occasions, 1 week apart. A semi-structured interview was followed in which participants were asked to describe their last trip to Greece. Participants were given the opportunity to talk as much as possible without being interrupted. For the participants with aphasia a second topic ("Tell me about your stroke") was made available for individuals who needed further prompting to reach the 300-word limit. Spontaneous speech samples were video recorded and transcribed verbatim.

Object and action naming. For the object and action naming tasks, the same sets of action and object pictures were administered in Greek and English. The order of language (Greek or English) was counterbalanced across the participants for each group separately. There was at least 1 week between the assessment of each of the two languages. The object naming task comprised 55 photographs in total, all designed to elicit one correct response. Similarly, action naming comprised 55 photographs designed to elicit one specific mono-transitive verb denoting one simple action. Participants were asked to name (in one word) the object or action represented in the photograph in the target language. Two examples in the target language were provided before testing. The stimulus question(s) was repeated once for participants who did not respond. If no response was given, the item was scored as incorrect. No time limits were placed and self-correction was allowed.

RESULTS

Spontaneous speech

The following lexical information was coded for 10 bilingual participants with aphasia and 10 controls: numbers of types and tokens of nouns, number of types and tokens of verbs, in both L1 and L2. This information is depicted for both groups of participants in Table 3. Furthermore, verb/noun diversity in L1 and L2 for both participant groups was determined by dividing the total number of verbs/nouns produced in spontaneous speech with the total number of verb/noun types to express a type-token ratio for each word class (see Bastiaanse & Jonkers, 1998). The results are depicted in Table 3. Individual results are provided in Appendix C.

An independent t-test between groups (participants with aphasia versus controls) revealed no significant differences when retrieving verbs in spontaneous speech in L1, $t(18) = 0.35$, ns, or in L2, $t(18) = 0.09$, ns. However, the bilingual participants with aphasia did differ significantly from controls in relation to noun production in spontaneous speech in L1, $t(18) = 2.53$, $p = < .05$, and in L2, $t(18) = 2.09$, $p = < .05$.

In addition, when verb and noun production (tokens) were investigated in bilingual participants with aphasia only, participants demonstrated a significant difference between languages for verbs, $t(9) = 2.78$, $p = < .05$, but not for nouns, $t(9) = 1.04$, ns. This same finding was also observed in the unimpaired control group for verbs, $t(9) = 5.24$, $p = < .05$, and nouns, $t(9) = 1.03$, ns. With regard to verb/noun diversity in spontaneous speech (expressed in type–token ratios), there was no significant difference between the two groups with respect to verbs in L1, $t(18) = 0.09$, ns, whereas a significant difference was observed in L2, $t(18) = 2.39$, $p = < .05$. This result showed that bilingual participants with aphasia had greater difficulty than the control group in producing different kinds of verbs in their second language (English) but not in their native language (Greek). On the other hand, when noun diversity was compared between the two groups there was a significant difference of diversity in L1 noun production, $t(18) = 3.47$, $p = < .05$, but not in L2, $t(18) = 1.69$, ns, revealing that bilingual participants with aphasia experienced less difficulty producing nouns in L2 than in L1 (see Table 4).

In addition there was a non-significant difference between languages for overall verb diversity, $t(9) = 1.09$, ns, and noun diversity, $t(9) = 1.03$, ns, in the spontaneous speech of the bilingual participants with aphasia. The same finding was apparent in the control group for verbs, $t(9) = 2.21$, ns, and nouns, $t(9) = 1.33$, ns.

TABLE 3

Noun/verb types and tokens produced by bilingual participants with aphasia and control participants in spontaneous speech in L1 and L2

	Noun types		Noun tokens		Verb types		Verb tokens	
	L1	L2	L1	L2	L1	L2	L1	L2
Aphasia								
Mean	26.6	26.3	41.3	39.1	34.8	24.8	57.6	45.1
SD	7.9	6.2	8.4	8.9	11.1	8.1	9.1	7.8
Controls								
Mean	41.0	36.5	52.9	49.7	35.2	30.2	59.0	45.5
SD	10.7	11.7	11.8	13.3	6.8	8.3	9.1	12.6

TABLE 4
Mean type–token ratios for noun and verb production in spontaneous speech for the bilingual
participants with aphasia and controls in L1 and L2

	Nouns		Verbs	
	L1	L2	L1	L2
Aphasia	0.64	0.68	0.60	0.55
Controls	0.77	0.73	0.60	0.65

Action–object naming and verb–noun retrieval in spontaneous speech

Individual results for action and object naming tests for participants with aphasia with mean performance of the control group are shown in Appendix D (Kambanaros & van Steenbrugge, 2006). Correlations based on spontaneous speech performance of the 10 participants and their corresponding action naming scores were calculated. The correlation between action/verb naming and number of verbs in spontaneous speech was not significant in either language: L1 (rho = 0.45, ns), L2 (rho = 0.28, ns). In contrast, the correlation between the results on the object/noun naming task and the number of nouns in spontaneous speech was significant in L1 (rho = 0.82, $p < .05$) but not in L2 (rho = 0.51, ns).

The correlation between action/verb naming performances and the diversity of verbs in spontaneous speech (the type–token ratio) was significant in L1 (rho = 0.65, $p < .05$) but not in L2 (rho = 0.31, ns). Furthermore, the correlation between object/noun naming performances and the diversity of nouns in spontaneous speech (the type–token ratio) failed to reach significance in either language: L1 (rho = 0.54, ns) and L2 (rho = 0.62, $p = .058$).

DISCUSSION

The present study sought to explore findings in the monolingual literature with regards to verb and noun processing in (fluent) anomic aphasia, and examine whether elicitation procedure, or context, had an effect on grammatical word class retrieval (Berndt, Burton, Haendiges, & Mitchum, 2002) in bilingual speakers with anomia. These issues were addressed by investigating whether grammatical class deficits in late bilingual individuals with anomia were specific to L1 (Greek) or L2 (English) in spontaneous speech and naming. The relevance of studying bilingual aphasia was to determine whether differences in verb and noun processing are an artefact of differences in language type. In addition, understanding this phenomenon has implications for models of bilingual lexical processing in unimpaired and bilingual participants with aphasia in more than one language.

The quantitative results from various language tasks were also compared with a control group of unimpaired bilingual speakers who were matched for age, gender, and education. When spontaneous speech samples from both languages were analysed for number (tokens) of verbs in spontaneous speech, fluent participants with anomia showed no significant differences compared to controls in retrieving verbs in either L1 (Greek) or L2 (English). This finding of a contextual influence in word retrieval lends support to other research showing that verb-impaired bilingual participants with fluent aphasia are able to produce a normal number (or more) of verbs in spontaneous speech compared to unimpaired controls (Luzzatti et al., 2006), despite difficulties on action picture naming (see also Bastiaanse & Jonkers, 1998, who reported similar results for monolingual Dutch speakers with anomia). It seems verb retrieval for late bilingual Greek–English participants in this study was facilitated by sentence frames (Berndt & Haendiges, 2000; Marshall et al., 1998) available in connected speech and facilitated by semantic and pragmatic factors in both L1 (Greek) and L2 (English). This pattern reflects what is typically described for participants with aphasia, i.e., no impairments in applying grammatical operations to build a sentence since the level of breakdown in anomia is not in the grammatical encoder (Levelt, 1989).

With regard to the different types of verbs—that is, the diversity (type–token ratios) produced in spontaneous speech—the results reveal a language-specific effect. Participants with aphasia had more difficulty than controls in producing different kinds of verbs in their second language (English) as revealed by their reduced type–token ratio results, but not in their native language (Greek). It is likely that English proficiency could explain this result, since L2 was more susceptible to word retrieval impairments in this study, as revealed by lower performance of participants with aphasia on all language tasks in English. Given that this group of participants with aphasia acquired English as a second language informally (usually in their job) and in young adulthood, it is possible the association or connections between lemmas and lexemes was weaker in L2 than in L1. This is based on the assumption that, when one learns a second language after childhood, both lexical and conceptual connections are active during bilingual word processing, but the strength of the connections or associations differs according to the relative dominance of L1 over L2 (or vice versa) as well as the language proficiency in L2 (Kroll & Stewart, 1994).

The finding for L2 (English) is in line with reports that (monolingual) fluent speakers with aphasia (across languages) produce fewer diverse verbs in connected speech or use a smaller set of verbs when compared to control subjects (Bastiaanse, Edwards & Kiss, 1996; Bastiaanse & Jonkers, 1998; Berndt et al., 1997a; Edwards & Bastiaanse, 1998). In contrast, results in L1 (Greek) are similar to findings reported by Luzzatti et al. (2006) for their verb-impaired fluent monolingual Italian participants who presented with a similar type-count analysis as the unimpaired controls.

On the other hand, when spontaneous speech samples in both languages were analysed for number (tokens) of nouns, participants with aphasia differ significantly from controls in relation to noun production in spontaneous speech—in Greek (L1) and in English (L2). Participants with aphasia demonstrated poorer retrieval of nouns in spontaneous speech in both their languages compared to the control group. This significant difference in relation to context for nouns was surprising given the overall verb impairment in the participants with aphasia based on the results of the action and object naming tests in L1 and L2. A different explanation may be related to strategies employed by participants with aphasia when retrieving nouns in naming vs connected speech based on resource demands for the two tasks and lexical-external variables (Pashek & Tompkins, 2002). It may be easier to retrieve object names from a static picture (intact perceptual encoding) whereas noun retrieval in spontaneous speech may be hindered by lexical-external variables related to macrostructural features such as thematic coherence (Glosser, 1991). Moreover, participants with aphasia do have overall word-finding difficulties. From scores on the object naming test it is clear that noun retrieval in isolation is far from perfect suggesting the results from spontaneous speech are not unexpected.

Furthermore, when noun diversity was compared between groups there was a significant difference of diversity in (Greek) L1 noun production but not in (English) L2, revealing that the participants with aphasia experienced less difficulty producing different kinds of nouns in L2 than in L1. It is possible to attribute this difference in L1 to bilingual participants reliance on verbs in L1 spontaneous speech production as revealed by the greater verb count and diversity of verbs in spoken Greek.

To determine any potential task-related difference in verb and noun retrieval, correlations were used to compare action and object naming performances on picture naming tasks with production of verbs and nouns in spontaneous speech. There was no significant correlation between the two tasks for verb retrieval in either Greek (L1) or English (L2). The results for this group of late bilingual participants are in line with similar findings for monolingual anomic speakers of Dutch (Edwards & Bastiaanse, 1998; Jonkers & Bastiaanse, 1998) and English (Edwards & Bastiaanse, 1998). In contrast, the correlation between results on the object naming task and the number of nouns produced in spontaneous speech was significant in Greek (L1) but not English (L2). The fact that naming static pictures of object names was easier in Greek than retrieving nouns in spontaneous speech could be related to factors described above in relation to number (tokens) of nouns produced in L1 spontaneous speech. In addition, correlations were performed between action and object naming performances and the diversity of verbs and nouns produced in spontaneous speech (the type–token ratios) for both languages. A language-specific effect was seen for verbs with a significant correlation between action naming and diversity of verb types in spontaneous speech for Greek (L1) but not English (L2). This result was foreseeable, given the normal number (tokens) of verbs and high type–token ratios in Greek (L1) spontaneous speech. Furthermore, the correlation between object naming and diversity of nouns in spontaneous speech (the type–token ratio) was not significant in Greek (L1) or English (L2).

Current models of naming are unable to describe the complexity of retrieval processes in connected speech (Berndt et al., 1997a) and performances in the object and action naming tasks in this study were not predictive of word-finding abilities in spontaneous speech for either nouns or verbs in L1 and L2. Furthermore, the marked differences between tasks such as performance on naming (actions and objects) in isolation and the production of verbs/nouns in spontaneous speech are not consistent with previous findings that suggest a direct (one-to-one) relationship between the two tasks (Berndt et al., 1997a; Herbert, Hickin, Howard, Osborne, & Best, 2007) but are more in tune with studies demonstrating different retrieval performance according to retrieval context for monolingual speakers with fluent aphasia in English (Berndt & Haendiges, 2000; Mayer & Murray, 2003; Pashek & Tompkins, 2002; Williams & Canter, 1987; Zingeser & Berndt. 1988) and Italian (Luzzatti et al., 2006).

The finding with regard to verb retrieval supports the suggestion made by Bastiaanse and Jonkers (1998), namely single-word naming performance (for verbs) is not necessarily representative of performance in conversation in aphasia. Even though picture naming remains the standard pointer of word retrieval ability in the monolingual and bilingual aphasia studies presented in this research, naming scores can both underestimate (e.g., action naming<verb naming in spontaneous speech

and also overestimate (e.g., object naming>noun retrieval in connected speech) word retrieval performances in connected speech as revealed by the results of this study.

Part of the difficulty in pinning down word retrieval deficits in aphasia as related to context may be due to a wide range of influences, some less obvious than others. There is no doubt that representations within the lexicon affect word class retrieval; that is, the formal properties of nouns and verbs (e.g., conceptual-semantic and morpho-syntactic properties, range of syntactic functions, distribution). However, it is possible that lexicon-external mechanisms not typically considered as operations at the macrostructural (discourse) level may play a role in retrieval context differences for verb/nouns in conversation for individuals with aphasia and as such, need to be further addressed (Levelt, Roelofs, & Meyer, 1999).

Other theories assume that verbs and nouns are stored in independent subsystems or storage modules, possibly with distinct neural substrates/pathways for retrieving the phonological (or orthographic) form (Caramazza & Hillis, 1991; Manning & Warrington, 1996; Miceli et al., 1988; Miozzo et al., 1994)[2] and are affected to a different extent after brain damage; that is, brain damage can selectively spare or impair either class. However, the different results based on the two different tasks (verbs worse than nouns in naming, verbs better than nouns in spontaneous speech) in both languages challenges this proposition.

The fact that similar patterns of noun–verb dissociation are seen in connected speech and picture naming tasks in both languages suggests this dissociation is not specific to either Greek (L1) or English (L2), but is likely to arise from more universal conceptual and/or linguistic properties that differentiate words belonging to the two grammatical categories. As such, it leads to processing variances when retrieving words of the two grammatical categories.

Given the diagnosis of anomic aphasia for the bilingual participants, the impairments in both languages are likely the result of a greater difficulty accessing the (morpho-) phonological representation or lexemes given that the syntactic information is also important during the activation of its morphological representation. Moreover, it is also possible that grammatical words are affected differently by semantic and syntactic characteristics during morpho-phonological processing (Bachoud-Levi & Dupoux, 2003; Edwards, 2002). According to Marshall (2003, p. 77):

> [t]hese different accounts need not be mutually exclusive. Rather, it seems that individuals show word class effects for different reasons. In other words, despite some common symptoms, people with word class effects are probably a very disparate group, a situation which is not at all unfamiliar in aphasia.

CONCLUSION

Overall, bilingual anomic individuals demonstrated no significant difficulties producing verbs in connected speech in either language. However, they did produce significantly more verbs in their native Greek. By contrast, they demonstrated more difficulty in producing nouns in spontaneous speech in both languages. When

---

[2] Others suggest that nouns and verbs are organised in a single semantic system (Moss, DeMornay Davies, Jeppeson, McLellan, & Tyler, 1998).

compared to their matched controls they produced a significantly smaller variety of verbs in their second language (English) but had more difficulty with the production of diverse nouns in their native language (Greek). Nevertheless, similar patterns of performance for both languages on tests of verb and noun retrieval across contexts were reported suggesting that despite significant differences in the morphological complexity of the two languages spoken by bilingual participants, conceptual and lexical representations of the two languages may share cerebral principles governing their organisation.

Results of the current study highlight the need to explore the under-researched area of grammatical word class breakdown in more detail for bilingual participants with aphasia. In particular, researchers need to examine closely (1) bilingual speakers' knowledge of verbs/nouns in their two languages, (2) word-finding difficulties for verbs/nouns in naming and in connected speech in both languages spoken by bilingual individuals, (3) measures and interpretations of the findings. However, the key results from this study are the following. For a group of late bilingual speakers of Greek (L1) and English (L2), there was (i) an effect of different contexts (picture naming versus conversation) on retrieval across grammatical word classes (nouns versus verbs) and (ii) similar patterns of performance in two languages that are fundamentally different in their lexical make-up and morphological word-formation processes. Future studies might aim to capture different aspects by investigating the verb–noun dichotomy in languages with different underlying forms or participants with aphasia who have different types of bilingualism, e.g., early L2 acquisition. Nevertheless, the growing interest in bilingual aphasia makes the study of word retrieval deficits in speakers of two (or more) languages a subject ripe for further exploration.

REFERENCES

Bachoud-Levi, A. C., & Dupoux, E. (2003). An influence of syntactic and semantic variables on word form retrieval. *Cognitive Neuropsychology*, *20*(2), 163–188.

Basso, A., Razzano, C., Faglioni, P., & Zanobio, M. E. (1990). Confrontation naming, picture description and action naming in aphasic patients. *Aphasiology*, *4*, 185–195.

Bastiaanse, R. (1991). Retrieval of instrumental verbs in aphasia: An explorative study. *Clinical Linguistics and Phonetics*, *5*(4), 355–368.

Bastiaanse, R., Edwards, S., & Kiss, K. (1996). Fluent aphasia in three languages: Aspects of spontaneous speech. *Aphasiology*, *10*, 561–575.

Bastiaanse, R., & Jonkers, R. (1998). Verb retrieval in action naming and spontaneous speech in agrammatic and anomic aphasia. *Aphasiology*, *12*, 99–117.

Bates, E., Chen, S., Tzeng, O., Li, P., & Opie, M. (1991). The noun-verb problem in Chinese. *Brain and Language*, *41*, 203–233.

Berndt, R. S., Burton, M. W., Haendiges, A. N., & Mitchum, C. (2002). Production of nouns and verbs in aphasia: Effects of elicitation techniques. *Aphasiology*, *16*(1/2), 83–106.

Berndt, R. S., & Haendiges, A. N. (2000). Grammatical class in word and sentence production: Evidence from an aphasic patient. *Journal of Memory and Language*, *43*, 249–273.

Berndt, R. S., Haendiges, A. N., Mitchum, C. C., & Sandson, J. (1997a). Verb retrieval in aphasia: Relationship to sentence processing. *Brain and Language*, *56*, 107–137.

Berndt, R. S., Haendiges, A. N., & Wozniak, M. A. (1997b). Verb retrieval and sentence processing: Dissociation of an established symptom association. *Cortex*, *33*, 99–114.

Berndt, R. S., Mitchum, C. C., & Haendiges, A. N. (1997c). Verb retrieval in aphasia. 1. Characterizing single word impairments. *Brain and Language*, *56*, 68–106.

Breedin, S. D., Saffran, E. M., & Schwartz, M. F. (1998). Semantic factors in verb retrieval: An effect of complexity. *Brain and Language, 63*, 1–31.

Breen, K., & Warrington, E. K. (1994). A study of anomia: Evidence for a distinction between nominal and propositional language. *Cortex, 30*, 231–245.

Caramazza, A., & Hillis, A. (1991). Lexical organization of nouns and verbs in the brain. *Nature, 349*, 788–790.

Chen, S., & Bates, E. (1998). The dissociation between nouns and verbs in Broca's and Wernicke's aphasia: Findings from Chinese. *Aphasiology, 12*, 5–36.

Daniele, A., Giustolisi, L., Silveri, M. C., Colosimo, C., & Gainotti, G. (1994). Evidence for a possible neuroanatomical basis for lexical processing of nouns and verbs. *Neuropsychology, 32*, 1325–1341.

De Bleser, R., & Kauschke, C. (2002). Acquisition and loss of nouns and verbs: Parallel or divergent patterns? *Brain and Language, 83*, 176–178.

Edwards, S. (2002). Grammar and fluent aphasia. In E. Fava (Ed.), *Clinical linguistics theory and applications in speech pathology and therapy* (pp. 249–266). Amsterdam/Philadelphia: John Benjamins.

Edwards, S., & Bastiaanse, R. (1998). Diversity in the lexical and syntactic abilities of fluent aphasic speakers. *Aphasiology, 12*, 99–117.

Glosser, G. (1991). Patterns of discourse production among neurological patients with fluent language disorders. *Brain and Language, 40*, 67–88.

Goodglass, H., & Kaplan, E. (1983). *The assessment of aphasia and related disorders* (2nd ed.). Philadelphia: Lea & Febiger.

Herbert, R., Hickin, J., Howard, D., Osborne, F., & Best, W. (2007). Do picture-naming tests provide a valid assessment of lexical retrieval in conversation in aphasia? *Aphasiology, 22*(2), 184–203.

Hernandez, M., Cano, A., Costa, A., Sebastian-Galles, N., Juncadella, M., & Gascon-Bayarri, J. (2008). Grammatical category-specific deficits in bilingual aphasia. *Brain and Language, 107*(1), 68–80.

Hernandez, M., Costa, A., Sebastian-Galles, N., Juncadella, M., & Rene, R. (2006). The organisation of nouns and verbs in bilingual speakers: A case of bilingual grammatical category-specific deficit. *Journal of Neurolinguistics, 20*(4), 285–305.

Hillis, A., & Caramazza, A. (1995). The compositionality of lexical semantic representations: Clues from semantic errors in object naming. *Memory, 3*, 333–358.

Jensen, L. R. (2000). Canonical structure without access to verbs. *Aphasiology, 14*(8), 827–850.

Jonkers, R. (1998). *Comprehension and production of verbs in aphasic speakers*. Unpublished PhD thesis, Rijksuniversiteit Groningen, The Netherlands.

Jonkers, R., & Bastiaanse, R. (1996). The influence of instrumentality and transitivity on action naming in Broca's and anomic aphasia. *Brain and Language, 55*, 37–39.

Jonkers, R., & Bastiaanse, R. (1998). How selective are selective word class deficits? Two case studies of action and object naming. *Aphasiology, 12*(3), 245–256.

Kambanaros, M. (2003). Naming errors in bilingual aphasia: Implications for assessment and treatment. *Brain Impairment, 3*(2), 156–157.

Kambanaros, M. (2007). The trouble with nouns and verbs in Greek fluent aphasia. *Journal of Communication Disorders, 41*(1), 1–19.

Kambanaros, M., & van Steenbrugge, W. (2006). Noun and verb processing in Greek–English bilingual individuals with anomic aphasia and the effect of instrumentality and verb–noun name relation. *Brain and Language, 97*, 162–167.

Kim, M., & Thompson, C. K. (2000). Patterns of comprehension and production of nouns and verbs in agrammatism: Implications for lexical organization. *Brain and Language, 74*, 1–25.

Kohn, S., Lorch, M., & Pearson, D. (1989). Verb finding in aphasia. *Cortex, 25*, 57–69.

Kremin, H. (1994). Selective impairments of action naming: Arguments and a case study. *Linguistiche Berichte, 6*, 62–82.

Kremin, H., & Basso, A. (1993). Apropos the mental lexicon. In F. J. Stachowiak, R. De Bleser, G. Deloche, R. Kaschel, H. Kremin, & P. North, et al. (Eds.), *Developments in the assessment and rehabilitation of brain-damaged patients – Perspectives from a European concerted action*. Tübingen: Narr Verlag.

Kremin, H., & De Agostini, M. (1995). Impaired and preserved picture naming in two bilingual patients with brain damage. In M. Paradis (Ed.), *Aspects of bilingual aphasia* (pp. 101–110). New York: Elsevier.

Kroll, J. F., & Stewart, E. (1994). Category interference in translation and picture naming: Evidence for asymmetric connections between bilingual memory representations. *Journal of Memory and Language, 33*, 149–174.

Kucera, H., & Francis, N. W. (1970). *Computational analysis of present-day American English*. Providence, RI: Brown University Press.

Laine, M., Kujala, P., Niemi, J., & Uusipaikka, E. (1992). On the nature of naming difficulties in aphasia. *Cortex, 28*, 537–554.

Levelt, W. (1989). *Speaking*. Cambridge, MA: MIT Press.

Levelt, W. J. M., Roelofs, A., & Meyer, A. S. (1999). A theory of lexical access in speech production. *Behavioural and Brain Sciences, 22*, 1–75.

Luzzatti, C., Ingignoli, C., Crepaldi, D., & Semenza, C. (2006). Noun–verb dissociation in aphasia: Type/token differences in the analysis of spontaneous speech. *Brain and Language, 99*(1–2), 159–160.

Luzzatti, C., Raggi, R., Zonca, G., Pistarini, C., Contardi, A., & Pinna, G. D. (2002). Verb–noun double dissociation in aphasic lexical impairments: The role of word frequency and imageability. *Brain and Language, 81*, 432–444.

Manning, L., & Warrington, E. (1996). Two routes to naming: A case study. *Neuropsychologia, 34*(8), 809–817.

Marshall, J. (2003). Noun–verb dissociations – evidence from acquisition and developmental and acquired impairments. *Journal of Neurolinguistics, 16*(2–3), 67–84.

Marshall, J., Pring, T., & Chiat, S. (1998). Verb retrieval and sentence production in aphasia. *Brain and Language, 63*, 159–183.

Mayer, J. F., & Murray, L. L. (2003). Functional measures of naming in aphasia: Word retrieval in confrontation naming versus connected speech. *Aphasiology, 17*(5), 481–497.

McCann, C., & Edwards, S. (2002). Verb problems in fluent aphasia. *Brain and Language, 83*, 42–44.

McCarthy, R., & Warrington, E. (1985). Category specificity in an agrammatic patient: The relative impairment of verb retrieval and comprehension. *Neuropsychologia, 23*, 709–727.

Miceli, G., Silveri, C., Noncentini, U., & Caramazza, A. (1988). Patterns of disassociation in comprehension and production of nouns and verbs. *Aphasiology, 2*, 351–358.

Miceli, G., Silveri, C., Villa, G., & Caramazza, A. (1984). On the basis for the agrammatic's difficulty in producing main verbs. *Cortex, 20*(2), 207–220.

Miozzo, A., Soardi, M., & Cappa, S. F. (1994). Pure anomia with spared action naming due to a left temporal lesion. *Neuropsychologia, 32*(9), 1101–1109.

Moss, H. E., DeMornay Davies, P., Jeppeson, C., McLella, S., & Tyler, L. K. (1998). The relationship between knowledge of nouns and verbs in a category specific deficit for living things. *Brain and Language, 65*, 92–95.

Osman-Sagi, J. (1987). Action naming in Hungarian aphasic patients. *Neuroscience, 22*(suppl.), 5509.

Pashek, G. V., & Tompkins, C. A. (2002). Context and word class influences on lexical retrieval in aphasia. *Aphasiology, 16*(3), 261–286.

Sasanuma, S., & Park, H. S. (1995). Patterns of language deficits in two Korean–Japanese bilingual aphasic patients: A clinical report. In M. Paradis (Ed.), *Aspects of bilingual aphasia* (pp. 111–123). New York: Elsevier.

Shapiro, K., Shelton, J., & Caramazza, A. (2000). Grammatical class in lexical production and morphological processing: Evidence from a case of fluent aphasia. *Cognitive Neuropsychology, 17*(8), 665–682.

Silveri, M. C., & Di Betta, A. M. (1997). Noun–verb dissociations in brain-damaged patients: Further evidence. *Neurocase, 3*, 477–488.

Tsapkini, K., Jarema, G., & Kehayia, E. (2002). Regularity revisited: Evidence from lexical access of verbs and nouns in Greek. *Brain and Language, 81*, 1–3, 103–119.

Tsolaki, M. (1997). *The neuropsychological evaluation of the elderly* [translated title of the Greek book]. Thessaloniki.

Weber-Fox, C. M., & Neville, H. J. (1996). Maturational constraints on functional specializations for language processing: ERP and behavioural evidence in bilingual speakers. *Journal of Cognitive Neuroscience, 8*, 231–256.

Williams, S. E., & Canter, G. J. (1982). The influence of situational context on naming performance in aphasic syndromes. *Brain and Language, 17*, 92–106.

Williams, S. E., & Canter, G. J. (1987). Action-naming performance in four syndromes of aphasia. *Brain and Language, 32*, 124–136.

Zingeser, L., & Berndt, R. (1988). Grammatical class and context effects in a case of pure anomia: Implications for models of language production. *Cognitive Neuropsychology, 5*, 473–516.

Zingeser, L., & Berndt, R. S. (1990). Retrieval of nouns and verbs in agrammatism and anomia. *Brain and Language, 39*, 14–32.

APPENDIX A

Demographic characteristics of participants with bilingual aphasia, including their year of birth, mean number of years of formal education, mean age at arrival in Australia, mean number of years of living in Australia, and information on lesion site, aphasia type and years post onset.

Participant	Gender	Year of birth	Lesion	Years post onset	Previous occupation	Years of education	Age at migration	Years in Australia
BA 1	M	1928	L. CVA	7	Factory worker	3	22	52
BA 2	M	1918	L. cerebral infarct	5	Factory worker	2	31	53
BA 3	F	1936	*L. fronto-parietal CVA	1	Factory worker	1	22	44
BA 4	M	1943	L. parietal CVA	2	Restaurant owner	8	14	46
BA 5	F	1933	L. internal capsule infarct	5	Farmer	5	21	46
BA 6	M	1934	*L. thalamus and posterior limb of the internal capsule	2	Waiter	11	27	41
BA 7	M	1939	L. basal ganglia involving thalamus and external capsule	3	Taxi driver	6	16	47
BA 8	M	1928	L. basal ganglia	5	Factory worker	3	25	49
BA 9	M	1930	*L. thalamic-internal capsule infarct	2	Factory worker	6	32	40
BA 10	F	1929	L. external capsule	1	Seamstress	6	28	45
BA 11	F	1932	L. MCA CVA involving parietal lobe	2	Factory worker	2	29	39
BA 12	M	1930	L. CVA	5	Factory worker	5	25	47
Mean		70.5 yrs		3.6 yrs		4.8 yrs	24.3 yrs	45.8 yrs

BA = bilingual aphasia (note: all participants in this table were born in Greece and their school education took place in Greece). M = male; F = female; CVA = cerebral vascular accident; L = left; MCA = middle cerebral artery; information about the lesion sites was obtained from the participants' medical records and was based on CT., scans except those marked with an * who were diagnosed using MRI scans.

APPENDIX B

The mean performance of participants with aphasia and controls on the Greek and English versions of the BDAE.

	Aphasia	Aphasia	Controls	Controls
	Greek (L1)	English (L2)	Greek (L1)	English (L2)
BDAE ratings				
Severity	4–5	3–4	–	–
Melody	6.3	5.8	7.0	7.0
Phrase length	6.4	5.4	7.0	7.0
Articulatory agility	6.3	6.2	7.0	7.0
Grammatical form	6.2	5.1	7.0	7.0
Repetition	8.0	8.0	8.0	8.0
Paraphasias	6.3	5.7	7.0	7.0
Word finding	3.0	2.7	4.0	4.0
Auditory comprehension (percentile)	65.7	48.1	87.4	85.8
BDAE subtests				
Word discrimination	65.3	60.3	72.0	71.5
Body parts	15.3	12.3	16.3	17.6
Commands	12.3	8.6	14.8	13.8
Complex ideation	5.9	3.4	10.8	9.8
Responsive naming	23.7	20.6	30.0	29.5
Confrontation naming	89.9	78.9	111.8	109.3
Animal naming	7.8	5.6	18.0	15.3

APPENDIX C

Total number of verb tokens and verb types retrieved in spontaneous speech by participants with aphasia and controls in L1 and in L2.

	Verb tokens		Verb types	
	Greek (L1)	English (L2)	Greek (L1)	English (L2)
Aphasia				
BA 1	54	54	26	38
BA 3	58	55	42	38
BA 4	65	33	28	18
BA 6	69	46	50	28
BA 7	60	51	44	26
BA 8	59	41	45	27
BA 9	56	35	29	19
BA 10	35	52	13	18
BA 11	58	44	33	18
BA 12	62	40	38	18
Controls				
BC 1	60	45	39	30
BC 3	72	60	47	40
BC 4	50	47	32	32
BC 6	51	42	31	24
BC 7	59	44	32	30
BC 8	60	30	30	20
BC 9	46	33	27	24
BC 10	70	59	44	36
BC 11	69	65	40	45
BC 12	53	30	30	21

APPENDIX D

Results on the action and object naming tests for participants with aphasia and controls.

	Action naming		Object naming	
	Greek (L1)	English (L2)	Greek (L1)	English (L2)
Bilingual participants				
BA 1	86.1	57.2	87.8	58.9
BA 2	57.2	25.0	64.4	35.6
BA 3	73.9	64.4	80	66.1
BA 4	14.4	20.6	27.8	16.7
BA 5	60.6	30.6	62.2	58.9
BA 6	80.6	58.9	87.8	73.3
BA 7	73.9	55.0	82.2	76.1
BA 8	73.3	48.9	80.6	58.3
BA 9	77.2	53.3	72.2	64.4
BA 10	8.9	22.2	13.3	59.4
BA 11	81.7	61.1	77.2	66.7
BA 12	65.0	60.0	72.2	66.7
Mean ±SD	62.7 ± 25.3	46.4 ± 16.7	67.3 ± 23.4	67.3 ± 16.6
Controls				
Mean ±SD	100 ± 0	96.6 ± 3.9	100 ± 0	95.7 ± 4.6

APHASIOLOGY, 2010, 24 (2), 231–261

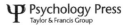

Semantic feature analysis treatment in Spanish–English and French–English bilingual aphasia

Swathi Kiran

Boston University, Boston, MA, USA

Patricia M. Roberts

University of Ottawa, Canada

Background: Edmonds and Kiran (2006) reported that training lexical retrieval in one language resulted in within-language and cross-language generalisation in three bilingual (English–Spanish) patients with aphasia.

Aims: The present experiment continues this line of research, repeating a similar procedure with new patients and examining a broader range of factors that may affect generalisation patterns.

Methods & Procedures: Four participants (two Spanish–English and two French–English speakers) with anomia post CVA received a semantic feature-based treatment aimed at improving naming of English or Spanish/French nouns. Using a multiple baseline design, generalisation to untrained semantically related and unrelated items in each language was measured during periods of therapy first in one language, then in the other.

Outcomes & Results: All patients improved their naming of the trained items in the trained language, although to varying degrees. Within-language generalisation to semantically related items occurred in two Spanish–English patients and one French–English patient. Cross-language generalisation to translations and semantically related items occurred only for one French–English patient.

Conclusions: The impact of the intervention is very clear. The semantic feature-based practice is linked to the gains made, and accounts for the predominance of semantic naming errors after treatment. Possible explanations for the different patterns of generalisation are considered in terms of the various factors including each patient's pre-stroke language proficiency, age of acquisition of each language, post-stroke level of language impairment, and type and severity of aphasia.

Keywords: Cross-language generalisation; Bilingual aphasia; Naming treatment; Semantic feature analysis; Aphasia.

Address correspondence to: Swathi Kiran, E-mail: kirans@bu.edu or Pat Roberts, proberts@uottawa.ca

This research was supported by an American Speech and Hearing Foundation New Investigator Grant to the first author. The authors thank Claudine Choquette, Mélanie Cohen, Anne Duff, and Deborah Kauffman for their work with the four patients. The translation advice of Linguistek and the University of Ottawa translation service was also very helpful. And, above all, we thank the four volunteers with aphasia who participated in the study over many hours of repetition and testing. Both authors contributed equally to this paper.

© 2010 Psychology Press, an imprint of the Taylor & Francis Group, an Informa business
http://www.psypress.com/aphasiology   DOI: 10.1080/02687030902958365

As clinicians face increasing numbers of bilingual patients and limited time for their treatment, the question of generalisation of treatment effects across languages in bilingual patients is an important one in aphasiology. On a clinical level, understanding why treatment in one language sometimes improves an untreated language, to varying degrees, and why it sometimes has little to no effect on the untreated language will help clinicians achieve maximum benefit for their patients in the minimum amount of time. To the extent that treatment effects generalise across languages, clinicians who do not speak the languages of their patients can nonetheless expect gains in these other languages following treatment in only one of the patient's languages (Roberts, 1998). To the extent that treatment gains are limited to the language of treatment, patients must receive treatment in all languages they need to use. On a theoretical level, studies of the effects of bilingual aphasia treatment can shed light on the structure and functioning of the bilingual language system and contribute evidence for or against various models of bilingual language processing.

Studies of cross-language generalisation have yielded a range of results. At times, the treated language improves more than the untreated one (i.e., limited cross-language generalisation), while other studies have found other patterns (see Roberts & Kiran, 2007, for a recent review of this literature).

One of the drawbacks of treatment case studies in bilingual aphasia is that they have only one or two patients and only one pair of languages in each study. As noted by Roberts and Kiran (2007), the variability inherent in both aphasia and bilingualism makes it difficult to interpret results obtained in therapy. Before drawing firm conclusions about the effects of various treatments and their implications for models of bilingualism, results must be shown to be consistent across patients and across studies. The primary aim of the present study is therefore to replicate and extend the work of Edmonds and Kiran (2006), by examining the results of treatment for anomia in new patients, including a new pair of languages (French–English).

Studies of normal bilingual individuals offer tests of models of lexical semantic representations and processing (de Groot, 1992; Dijkstra & Van Heuven, 2002; Green, 1998; Kroll & Stewart, 1994; Potter, So, von Eckardt, & Feldman, 1984). These models generally agree that bilingual individuals have a shared semantic/conceptual system and that there are separate lexical representations for the two languages. Some studies posit that the semantic system spreads its activation to lexical items in both languages regardless of the target language (for a recent review see Costa, La Heij, & Navarrete, 2006) with the size and direction of this spreading activation depending, to some extent, on age of acquisition and proficiency levels in each language (e.g., Silverberg & Samuel, 2004) as well as on the semantic similarity between the specific lexical items. To the— currently unknown—extent that this is true for patients with damaged language systems, generalisation of gains could occur across languages when semantic representations in one language are repeatedly activated during therapy.

For monolingual patients with aphasia, treatments based on models of lexical semantic processing that emphasise strengthening semantic information at the semantic/ conceptual level have been successful in facilitating generalisation to untrained semantically related items in some patients (Coelho, McHugh, & Boyle, 2000; Drew & Thompson, 1999; Kiran & Thompson, 2003). Therefore, training that strengthens or emphasises semantic features should increase the level of activation of trained items and of their semantically related neighbours, thereby facilitating generalisation to untrained semantically related items. It is also hypothesised that phonological representations of targets in both languages access a common semantic representation (de Groot, 1992), and semantic activation is thought to activate the phonological representations in both lexicons (e.g., Costa & Caramazza, 1999). Hence, the lexical forms that receive treatment in the target language will also activate translation equivalents in the non-target language, leading to improvement in these items as well.

In order to test the predictions outlined above, Edmonds and Kiran (2006) administered a semantic treatment to improve picture naming in English and Spanish and measured generalisation to translations of the treated words and to words semantically related to the target words, in each language. Results demonstrated within- and across-languages effects on generalisation that the authors interpreted as being related to pre-morbid language proficiencies. Participant 1, who claimed equal proficiency in English and Spanish, showed within-language general-isation in the trained language (Spanish) and some cross-language generalisation to the untrained language (English). The other two patients, who reported that English was their stronger language pre-stroke, showed cross-language generalisation from the trained language (Spanish) to the untrained language (English) but no within-language generalisation (to related words in Spanish). The results could be interpreted as showing that training the patient's weaker language may facilitate more cross-language generalisation than training their stronger language, but more patients need be examined to explore this very preliminary hypothesis.

One problem with interpreting the Edmonds and Kiran (2006) results in terms of reported pre-stroke level of bilingualism is the unknown validity of self-reports of proficiency. For example, their patient P1 claimed equal proficiency in English and Spanish for auditory comprehension, reading, and writing, and only slightly better Spanish for verbal expression. This profile is very surprising in someone who also stated that "she acquired English as an adult" (p. 732).

There are other factors that may influence the extent of cross-language generalisation. These include factors always present in studies of aphasia: the type and severity of the aphasia, lesion location (both macro and micro), and degree of impairment in each language. Additionally, factors related to bilingualism may be relevant: including domains of language use, age of acquisition, and the particular linguistic features of Spanish–English bilingualism. As noted by the authors, one limitation in the Edmonds and Kiran (2006) study was that only one of the three patients received therapy in both languages.

The present study examines the effects of a primarily semantic treatment on anomia in four patients and two language pairs (Spanish–English and French–English), exploring the same hypotheses as Edmonds and Kiran (2006). The theoretical foundations for these hypotheses are presented in detail in the 2006 paper. It was hypothesised that a primarily semantically based treatment would lead to:

1. gains on *trained items* in the *trained language* (e.g., English: *door*);
2. within-language generalisation to semantically related, not treated items (i.e., if *door* is practised in treatment, we expect improvement in *window*), if the gains in 1 are seen;
3. cross-language generalisation to the translations of the treated items (i.e., if *door* is practised in treatment, we expect improvement in *puerta* or in *porte*);
4. cross-language generalisation to items semantically related to the treated items in the untrained language (i.e., if *door* is practised, we expect improvement in the Spanish or French words for window: *ventana* or *fenêtre*).
5. No changes in semantically unrelated, "control words" in either language.

METHOD

Participants

Four bilingual women with aphasia (two English–Spanish and two French–English) were recruited from local area hospitals and stroke support groups in Austin, Texas, USA and Ottawa, Ontario, Canada. All participants met the following selection criteria: (a) diagnosis by a neurologist of a single stroke in the left hemisphere (encompassing the grey/white matter in and around the perisylvian area) confirmed by a CT/MRI scan; (b) onset of stroke at least 6 months prior to participation in the study; (c) right-handed prior to stroke; (d) adequate hearing, vision, and comprehension to engage fully in testing and treatment; (e) stable health status; (f) previous speech-language therapy had ended at least 1 month prior to starting the present study; (g) bilingual speakers of English and Spanish or English and French who reported regular use of both languages prior to their stroke; and (h) not able to speak any other language. See Table 1 for demographic details. None of the participants had diabetes. None reported any cognitive or communication problems prior to their stroke. All except P2 held full-time jobs prior to their stroke.

Language history, use patterns (Muñoz, Marquardt, & Copeland, 1999; Roberts & Shenker, 2007), and proficiency ratings were used to estimate pre-morbid proficiency in both languages. In addition to self-ratings, one bilingual family member familiar with the participant's language acquisition and use was also interviewed to corroborate information provided by the participants.

Participant 1 (P1)

Participant 1 had a single left hemisphere CVA 11 months prior to starting this study, and was diagnosed with severe expressive aphasia. Most of the therapy she received was in English. The patient reported that after her stroke she had more difficulty communicating in Spanish than in English. P1 presented with hemiparesis of her right hand and was diagnosed with verbal apraxia by the referring speech pathologist.

Language background. Participant 1 grew up in a predominantly Spanish-speaking home in Texas. She probably had some passive exposure to English before starting an English-language elementary school at age 5. As an adult she spoke in English and Spanish to her spouse, her children, and all relatives. However, she rated herself as being more proficient in English than in Spanish in her daily interactions with friends and family members. P1 spoke English with no Spanish accent.

Education and work history. P1 was educated in English and taught herself to read and write in Spanish up to high-school level. She worked as a clerk in a community education classroom for English as a second language. Therefore, prior to her stroke, she reported that she used English and Spanish relatively equally at work.

Participant 2 (P2)

Participant 2 had a single left hemisphere stroke approximately 6 months prior to the present study. She was diagnosed with receptive aphasia after her stroke and received therapy mainly in English. Although P2's aphasia resolved considerably in the first 6 months, she still presented with comprehension difficulties. She reported that the stroke affected both languages equally.

TABLE 1

Demographic data, language history, and language proficiency ratings across languages for all participants

	Demographic information				Language history and proficiency				
								Self-ratings (L1/L2) (1–7)	BPR
Pt	Sex	Age	Education	Aetiology	MPO	Family/social	Work	Reading/writing		
1	F	55	14 yrs?	Left MCA	11	Born in US. Began English at age 5. Spanish from birth. Married to bilingual Spanish speaker. Spoke both English and Spanish with children, siblings, with friends.	English: 50% Spanish 50% Clerk in community education for English as a second language	Educated in English Self-taught Spanish Read and wrote English and Spanish materials	Speech 6/7 Comp 6/7 Reading 4/7 Writing 4/7	.78 (English dominant)
2	F	87	12 years	Left MCA	6	Spanish only with parents, siblings, relatives, friends. English with grandchildren and other professionals.	50% English 50% Spanish Writer of Mexican fiction books	Educated in Spanish Wrote letters and lists in Spanish Learned and used English Read and wrote English and Spanish materials	Speak: 7/7 Comp: 7/7 Read: 7/7 Write: 7/7	1.0 (Equally proficient)
3	F	55	12 years	Left MCA	33	Grew up in bilingual environment but much more exposure to French than English. French spoken at home as child and mostly French as adult.	70% French; 30% English. Bank clerk, secretary; teacher's aide.	Education in French, except for 1 year of community college. Strong preference for French. Reads a little for pleasure, mostly in French	Speech 6/4 Comp 7/5 Reading 6/4 Writing 6/4	1.4 (French dominant)

(Continued)

TABLE 1
Continued

Demographic information					Language history and proficiency			Self-ratings (L1/L2) (1–7)	BPR
Pt	Sex	Age	Education	Aetiology	MPO	Family/social	Work	Reading/writing	
4	F	60	15 years	Left MCA	15	Grew up in French environment. Learned English from grade 3 onwards. Adult social life mostly in French	80% English 20% French; federal civil servant with administrative and training roles	Schooling primarily in French except university, which was in both languages. Avid reader of both languages with more exposure to English.	Speech 7/6 Comp 7/6 Reading 7/7 Writing 7/6	1.1 (Equally proficient/ French dominant)

MPO: Months Post Onset; E: English; S: Spanish; Comp: Comprehension; MCA: Middle Cerebral Artery; CVA: Cerebral Vascular Accident; BPR: Bilingual Proficiency Ratio.

Language background. P2 grew up in a predominantly Spanish-speaking environment in Mexico. Her exact age of immigration to the US is not known. As a child she spoke only Spanish with her parents, siblings, and relatives. As an adult she spoke English with most of her grandchildren and friends and other professionals. She reported that her linguistic environment as an adult was "100% bilingual" although she was more comfortable in Spanish than English. She spoke English with a strong Spanish accent.

Education and work history. P2 was educated in Spanish and took classes in English when she arrived in the US. Specific details about her education history are not available. She was a successful author, writing non-fiction books in Spanish and also worked in a Mexican art museum.

Participant 3(P3)

Participant 3 had a single left hemisphere CVA approximately 35 months prior to starting this study. She initially experienced quite severe aphasia and received therapy in French for approximately 3 months following her stroke. The aphasia resolved into a relatively mild aphasia, which seemed to affect both languages equally. French was her preferred/stronger language pre-stroke and remained so post-stroke. P3's initial hemiplegia had resolved into hemiparesis. However, she remained unable to use her right hand to write.

Language background. P3 reported that her family spoke French 90% of the time at home when she was a child. She reported some exposure to English at home, and through television prior to that, but the small rural Ontario community she grew up in was primarily French. She spoke English with a noticeable French accent, somewhat stronger than that of P4.

Education and work history. Language of instruction at school was French. P3 studied English as a subject beginning around age 10 or 11. She finished high school and took some courses at community college level but did not complete a diploma. She worked at various white-collar jobs, including bank teller (primarily in English) and, for the 10 years prior to her stroke, as a teaching assistant (primarily in French).

Participant 4 (P4)

Participant 4 experienced a left hemisphere stroke 14 months prior to starting this study. Initially she was diagnosed with moderate non-fluent aphasia with agrammatism, moderately severe verbal apraxia, and mild to moderate dysphagia. She received language therapy in English. Prior to beginning this study her aphasia was mild. Mild verbal apraxia remained, giving her speech a slightly slow and effortful quality and occasionally interfering with intelligibility. A mild French accent was present when she spoke English. Prior to this study she received individual speech-language therapy as an inpatient, then as an outpatient, primarily in English, with the most recent (group) treatment several months before the start of this study. She felt the stroke had affected the two languages about equally.

Language background. P4's family spoke French when she was a child in rural Ontario, near Ottawa. She reports beginning English classes in school around age 8 but had some exposure to English prior to age 8 through friends and neighbours. The language of instruction was French for elementary and high school, while university was in both languages.

Education and work history. P4 completed a bachelor's degree in psychology. At university, readings and classes were in both French and English. She worked at various white-collar jobs, primarily in the federal civil service. Prior to the stroke she had held an administrative and training position for many years where she used English 80% of the time and French 20% of the time.

To quantify pre-morbid language proficiencies, and to facilitate comparisons across patients, a bilingual proficiency ratio (BPR) was calculated by dividing the sum of the self-ratings in Spanish or French by the sum of the self-ratings in English: BPR=(Spanish/French comprehension+verbal expression+reading+writing)/(English comprehension+verbal expression+reading+writing). A BPR of 1 reflects equal language proficiency. Scores less than 1.0 reflect dominance in English, whereas scores greater than 1.0 reflect dominance in Spanish or French. Therefore, based on their self-reports, P1 was relatively English dominant (.78), P2 was equally proficient (1.0), P3 was relatively more dominant in French (1.4) and P4 was very close to balanced, but with a slight preference for French (1.1).

Language status after stroke

Prior to starting treatment, participants completed relevant portions of the *Western Aphasia Battery* (WAB; Kertesz, 1982) in English, several semantic and lexical subtests from the *Psycholinguistic Assessment of Language Processing in Aphasia* (PALPA; Kay, Lesser, & Coltheart, 1992) in English, the *Boston Naming Test* (BNT; Kaplan, Goodglass, & Weintraub, 2001) in both languages, and portions of the *Bilingual Aphasia Test* (BAT; Paradis, 1989) in both languages. Scores for the WAB, BNT, and the BAT cannot be interpreted as showing the relative severity of the aphasia in each language. However, they were administered to allow comparisons pre/post-therapy for each participant on each test. Summaries for each participant are provided in Tables 2 and 3.

Participant 1 was diagnosed with moderate aphasia characterised by nonfluent speech, relatively intact comprehension, and mild difficulties in repetition and naming based on the *WAB*. Performance on the two word-to-picture matching subtests of the PALPA revealed mild impairments. Her score on the BNT was 6/60 in Spanish and 34/60 in English. Performance on the various subtests of the BAT revealed an overall superior performance in English across receptive tests such as complex commands, judgement of words/nonwords, and semantic categories. The stronger performance in English was marked on tests that required verbal output such as naming, sentence construction, antonym distinction, reading text, and dictation. P1's comprehension in Spanish was much better than her production abilities.

Participant 2 had a moderate to severe aphasia characterised by fluent speech, impaired comprehension, and poor repetition and naming. Performance on the two word-to-picture matching subtests of the PALPA revealed moderate impairments. Performance on the BNT revealed severe naming deficits in both languages (5/60 in English and 3/60 in Spanish). Performance on the various subtests of the BAT revealed similar performance in English and Spanish on receptive tests such as pointing, semicomplex commands, grammaticality judgement, and judgement of

TABLE 2
Pre- and post-language performance on tests administered in English only: WAB (Kertesz, 1982)
and PALPA (Kay et al., 1992)

Test	Participant 1		Participant 2		Participant 3		Participant 4	
	Pre-tx	Post-tx	Pre-tx	Post-tx	Pre-tx	Post-tx	Pre-tx	Post-tx
Western Aphasia Battery (WAB)								
Spontaneous speech	11	12	14	16	15	15	16	16
Auditory comprehension	9.2	8.9	4.1	5.6	9.8	NA	8.9	NA
Repetition	7.1	6.4	2.3	2.9	9.5	NA	8.6	NA
Naming	7.6	7.7	4.0	5.4	7.2	7.9	8.2	NA
PALPA								
Spoken Word–Picture Matching (%)	90	90	80	70	90	NA	98	NA
Written Word–Picture Matching (%)	90	92.5	87.5	90	98	NA	98	NA
Auditory Synonym Judgements (%)	72	75	48	45	NA	NA	NA	NA
Written Synonym Judgements (%)	85	77	90	66.7	87	NA	NA	NA

NA indicates not administered.

words/nonwords. However, performance in English was superior to Spanish on subtests involving reading and verbal output.

Participant 3 displayed a mild anomic aphasia, with auditory comprehension superior to verbal expression, good repetition abilities, and mild to moderate naming deficits in both languages. She obtained near perfect scores on the PALPA subtests examining semantic processing. BNT scores were lower in English (22/60) than in French (39/60). On the BAT she showed some difficulty with syntactic structures. P3's performance was generally high in both languages, however relatively superior performance was observed for French on semantic categories, judgement of real words/nonwords, and semantic acceptability.

Participant 4 displayed a mild nonfluent aphasia characterised by relatively intact auditory and reading comprehension, good repetition abilities, mild agrammatic tendencies in spontaneous speech, and mild to moderate naming deficits in both languages. Performance on the two subtests of the PALPA revealed relatively normal performance. Performance on the BNT revealed mild naming impairments in English (42/60) and in French (43/60). Likewise she displayed mild deficits on various subtests of the BAT that included judgement of real/non words, repetition, semantic categories, semantic antonyms, synonyms, naming, and reading. In verbal fluency she performed better on semantic categories than on phonological ones. Overall, this patient demonstrated milder impairments than the three other participants, in both languages.

Stimuli

Five stimulus sets were created for each patient. The first set (English Set 1) consisted of picturable English nouns. French or Spanish Set 1 was the translation of English

TABLE 3
Performance selected sub-tests of Bilingual Aphasia Test before and after treatment

	P1 PRE-TX		P1 POST-TX		P2 PRE-TX		P2 POST-TX		P3 PRE-TX		P3 POST-TX		P4 PRE-TX		P4 POST-TX	
Task	E %	S %	E %	S %	E %	S %	E %	S %	E %	F %	E %	F %	E %	F %	E %	F %
Semi-complex Commands (10 points)	90	70	100	60	50	60	30	60	100	100	NA	NA	NA	NA	NA	NA
Complex Commands (20 points)	100	55	55	60	15	5	25	5	NA	80	NA	NA	85	NA	NA	NA
Semantic Categories (5 points)	80	40	80	80	20	0	60	40	80	100	NA	80	80	80	80	80
Synonyms (5 points)	100	80	100	60	20	0	0	0	100	100	NA	100	80	80	80	NA
Antonyms I (5 points)	100	60	100	40	20	0	20	0	80	80	NA	60	80	80	80	100
Antonyms II (5 points)	40	40	40	40	40	40	20	40	80	60	NA	60	80	80	90	80
Grammaticality Judgement (10 points)	50	70	70	50	50	60	50	40	80	100	NA	NA	80	80	90	80
Semantic Acceptability (10 points)	40	30	100	80	40	50	80	60	90	90	NA	NA	90	90	90	80
Repetition (30 points)	77	67	77	87	13	37	37	37	93	100	NA	NA	93	100	90	97
Judgment of words/nonwords (30 points)	90	73	97	90	70	60	67	73	87	100	NA	NA	87	93	80	97
Series (automatics) (3 points)	33	NA	0	0	0	0	33	67	NA	100	NA	NA	100	100	NA	NA
Naming (19 points)	100	26	100	32	25	25	50	25	NA	100	NA	NA	90	100	NA	NA
Semantic Opposites (10 points)	40	NA	30	10	0	0	60	10	NA	100	NA	NA	NA	80	70	90
Reading Words (10 points)	90	80	100	80	90	40	100	100	NA	100	NA	NA	100	100	NA	NA

E = English, S = Spanish, F = French.

Set 1. For each item in English Set 1 a semantically related category coordinate was included in English Set 2. French/Spanish Set 2 was a translation of English Set 2. Unrelated words made up Set 3, a control set. All words were non-cognates (defined as <50% overlap in phonemes). For P1 and P2 it was possible to find 15 words for Sets 1 and 2, providing a larger data set with which to measure changes during treatment. For P3 and P4 this was not feasible, so lists of 10 items were used, as in the Edmonds and Kiran study. See the appendix for lists of the stimuli used with each patient.

We attempted to match for perceived and written word frequency and for word length across the five lists, but the primary criterion was the patient's inability to name these pictures during baseline testing. The English words were verified in Francis and Kucera (1982), Thorndike and Lorge, and Brown at the MRC database site (http://www.psych.rl.ac.uk/MRC_Psych_Db.html). Spanish word frequency values were obtained from published norms (Juilland & Chang-Rodriguez, 1964). None of the published databases consulted contained word frequencies for all French words: Baudot (1992); Frantext (http://www.frantext.fr/noncateg.htm); Lexique 3 (www.lexique.org). Furthermore, homonyms/homographs used for all four participants were not listed separately (e.g., *bit*, *bolt*, *button*, *leg*, *counter*, *mouth* in English; *volet*, and *macaron*, in French). Therefore, valid word frequency values for all stimuli could not be obtained.

Ratings of semantic relatedness for the stimuli for P1 and P2 were based on previous studies (Edmonds & Kiran, 2006; Kiran & Lebel, 2007), using a 4-point scale. For P1 and P2, the mean ratings for semantic related pairs were 2.2 and 2.2 respectively. Ratings for semantic relatedness for stimuli for P3 and P4 were obtained from 19 naive judges on a 5-point scale. The means were 2.2 for P3 and 2.0 for P4. See the appendix for the stimulus lists. Colour pictures were chosen from Art Explosion Software® (NOVA Inc), and from C-O-L-O-U-R library photos from Communication Skill Builders. For *clasp*, *button*, and *glasses case*, the actual objects were used.

Development of semantic features for treatment

As in Edmonds and Kiran (2006), we developed a set of 12 yes/no questions for each target word similar to the approach of semantic feature analysis treatment, (Boyle, 2004; Boyle & Coehlo, 1995; Coelho et al., 2000). For six questions the answer was "yes" and for six it was "no". Questions for each item focused on: (1) the superordinate category (e.g., *fruit*; *insect*); (2) function or common use; (3) general characteristic "is a" (e.g., *is sweet*; *is made of metal*); (4) physical characteristic (e.g., *has skin/peel*; *has wings*); (5) typical location; (6) a personal association for each patient (*reminds me of …*). The associations were worked out with each patient in the first one or two sessions, with assistance from the clinician as needed.

Design

The experimental design was single-participant experimental across multiple behaviours and participants. All participants received three initial baseline sessions or enough testing sessions to find the required number of stimuli that the patient was consistently unable to name, in both languages. Treatment then began on one set of items in one language (e.g., English set 1). The remaining three sets of stimuli

(English set 2, French set 1, and French set 2) and the control items were verified after every second treatment session. For details about the order of treatment, see Table 4. The language of the first block of treatment was determined prior to recruiting the participants and was counterbalanced across participants. The goal was for patients to reach 80% accuracy in naming pictures in two of three consecutive sessions. If this level was not reached after 20 treatment sessions, treatment on that set of targets stopped. Subsequently, treatment was shifted to the semantically related set in the untrained language (e.g., if *shark* was trained in English then *ballena* was trained in Spanish).

Baseline measures

Baseline testing took place over several sessions, alternating which language was tested first and varying the order of stimuli each time. For the baseline and treatment probes, responses were considered correct if they were the expected (standard) name or a regional or slang term in wide use. Self-corrected responses were scored as correct. Minor apraxic or dysarthric errors were disregarded, except where a substituted phoneme resulted in a different word (e.g., *dog/bog*). All responses were coded into one of 10 categories. These were: (a) no response, (b) neologism or perseveration (defined as a repetition of a word at least three times within the same session), (c) unrelated word with no semantic or phonemic relationship to the target word, (d) phonemic error in target language (e.g., English – *pader* for *spider*), (e) semantic error in target language (e.g., English – *cabbage* for *radish*), (f) circumlocution, (g) mixed, semantic, and phonemic error (e.g., English *pur* for *wallet*), (h) phonemic error in nontarget language (e.g., *hooka* for *gancho* in Spanish); in some cases this error type corresponds to what other authors have called "false cognates" (e.g., Roberts & Deslauriers, 1999), (i) semantic error in nontarget language (e.g., *mesa* in Spanish for *chair*) and (j) correct response in nontarget language (e.g., *gato* in Spanish for *cat*).

For P1 it was difficult to settle on a set of items that were impaired in English and in Spanish, for two reasons. The patient was much more impaired in Spanish than in English naming, and her naming scores in English improved during baseline testing. Therefore after two attempts at finding stimuli she could not name in both English and Spanish, the focus shifted to finding items she was unable to name in Spanish. Consequently, P1's naming accuracy during baseline is higher in English than in

TABLE 4
Order of language and stimulus trained for each participant in the study

Participant	Language	Stimulus set trained
P1	1. Spanish	Spanish set 1
P2	1. English	English set 1
	2. Spanish	Spanish set 2
P3	1. French	French set 1
	2. English	English set 2
P4	1. English	English set 1
	2. French	French set 2

Spanish. Both P3 and P4 tended to improve during the baseline phase, which meant it was difficult to find sets of non-cognate words that they were consistently unable to name in both languages and for which clear pictures and a suitable semantically related word, also consistently failed, in both languages were available. Some words were eliminated as potential stimuli if the patient indicated that she did not recognise and/or would not have known the name pre stroke. Both women reported that sometimes the word for a picture they were unable to name during testing suddenly "came back" after testing, allowing them to correctly name that item in the next session. Sometimes this occurred before leaving the testing room. They also asked family members to provide names between sessions. For these reasons, the stimuli for each French–English participant included one pair that had weaker semantic relatedness than the preset minimum of 2.5/5 and three pairs that were closer to being cognates than optimal.

Treatment

Each set of target items was practised using a seven-step semantic feature analysis treatment method (Boyle & Coehlo, 1995; Edmonds & Kiran, 2006; Haarbauer-Krupa, Moser, Smith, Sullivan, & Szekeres, 1985) with the following characteristics: (1) the patient attempted to name the picture and was told if their answer was correct or not; (2) the clinician named the object; (3) the clinician placed the printed name of the picture on or below the picture; (4) the patient read a short sentence or phrase describing one of 12 semantic features of the object; (5) then sorted them into piles/groups of correct/incorrect features; (6) the picture was turned over for P1 and P2, but was left visible for P3 and P4 and the participants were asked the same 12 yes/no questions regarding these features (e.g., *Is it a fruit? Is it found on the roof?*); and (7) the patient named the picture again. Even if the participant named the picture correctly in Step 1, the whole procedure was followed. For the first sessions the clinician explained what each question was about: category name, function, etc., to make patients aware of the structure of the therapy.

Treatment probes

Every second session began with the administration of probes to measure progress on the target words and generalisation within and across languages to the related words and the control set of words. The language first assessed alternated from one probe session to the next. Responses to naming probes are the primary dependent measure for P1 and P2. For P3 and P4, because of the rapid improvement, their scores during treatment sessions are the dependent measures during the treatment phase in each language.

Data analysis

Effect sizes (ES) were calculated comparing the mean of all data points in the treatment and maintenance phases to the baseline mean divided by the standard deviation of baseline (Beeson & Robey, 2006; Busk & Serlin, 1992). When there was no variation in the baseline (e.g., accuracy was at 0% across the three baselines), the zero variance value was replaced with the mean variance of other baseline phase data for the same individual as recommended by Beeson and Robey (2006). Data from the follow-up phase were not included in the analysis. When treatment was shifted to the second language, the data preceding the onset of treatment were included within the baseline phase for that condition for that participant. Finally, because the French–English treatment comprised fewer sessions than the Spanish–English treatment, effect sizes for the generalisation (non-trained and control items) are calculated over the entire period and not specific to each treatment phase. Based on comparable naming treatment studies in aphasia, an ES of 4.0 was considered small, 7.0 was considered medium, and 10.1 was considered large (Beeson & Robey, 2006).

Reliability

All baseline and probe sessions were recorded on audiotape and/or videotape and scored by two different individuals. Point-to-point agreement was ≥90% across all sessions. Discrepancies were resolved by repeated listening to the tapes. Scoring of regional terms and decisions about acceptable synonyms were made after consulting dictionaries, other bilingual speakers, and professional translators.

RESULTS

Naming accuracy

Results for each patient are displayed in Figures 1 to 4. For reasons discussed above, data for P3 and P4 are their naming scores during the treatment phase. For P1 and P2, data are their naming scores during the weekly probes.

Participant 1

P1 was trained in Spanish (her weaker language). After three baseline sessions, naming of set 1 improved to a high of 53%, which did not meet criterion despite the effect size of 7.4. Concomitant changes were observed in the semantically related but untrained Spanish set 2 (ES = 1.2), which improved to a high of 47%. English translations (English set 1) of the trained items also improved to a high of 70% (ES = 2.2), continuing the rising baselines pattern pre-therapy. Performance on untrained, English, semantically related items (English set 2) showed a slight improvement but performance fluctuated between 40 and 67% (ES = 2.3). Because performance on both English sets improved during Spanish treatment to reach over 60% accuracy, treatment was not provided in English.

Performance on the English unrelated control items showed an improvement from 33% to a high of 83% (ES = 3.5). Although this change appears to be quite dramatic it is amplified because there were only five items in this set. No changes were observed in the Spanish unrelated control words (ES = 0.2).

Participant 2

P2 was trained first in English and then in Spanish. On English set 1 performance improved to 66% (ES = 10.1) after nine sessions. Performance on the semantically related items in English (English set 2) showed a trend of improvement (from 6% to a maximum score of 40%). Performance on the Spanish translations of the items trained in English (Spanish set 1) also improved slightly (from 0% to 27%). No changes were observed in Spanish set 2. Treatment then began with this set as the target words.

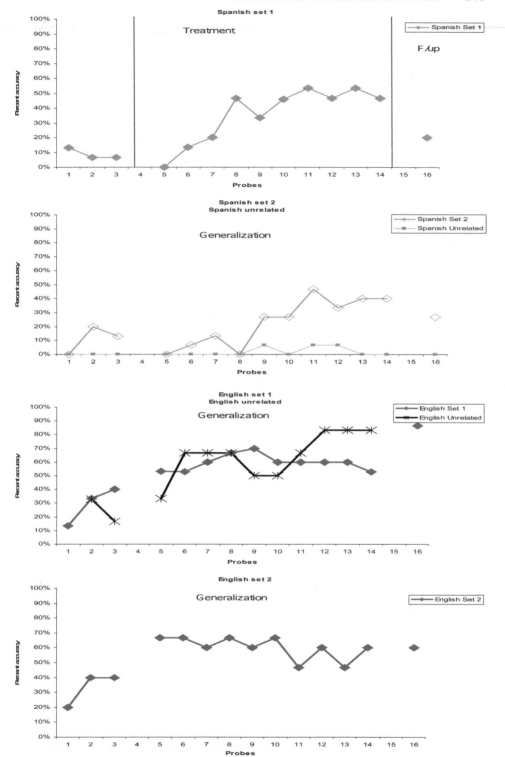

Figure 1. Naming accuracy for Participant 1 on Spanish set 1 (trained) and Spanish set 2 (semantically related to set 1), English set 1 (translations of Spanish set 1) and English set 2 (semantically related translations). Control (unrelated) items in English and Spanish are illustrated in the same graph as the generalisation items.

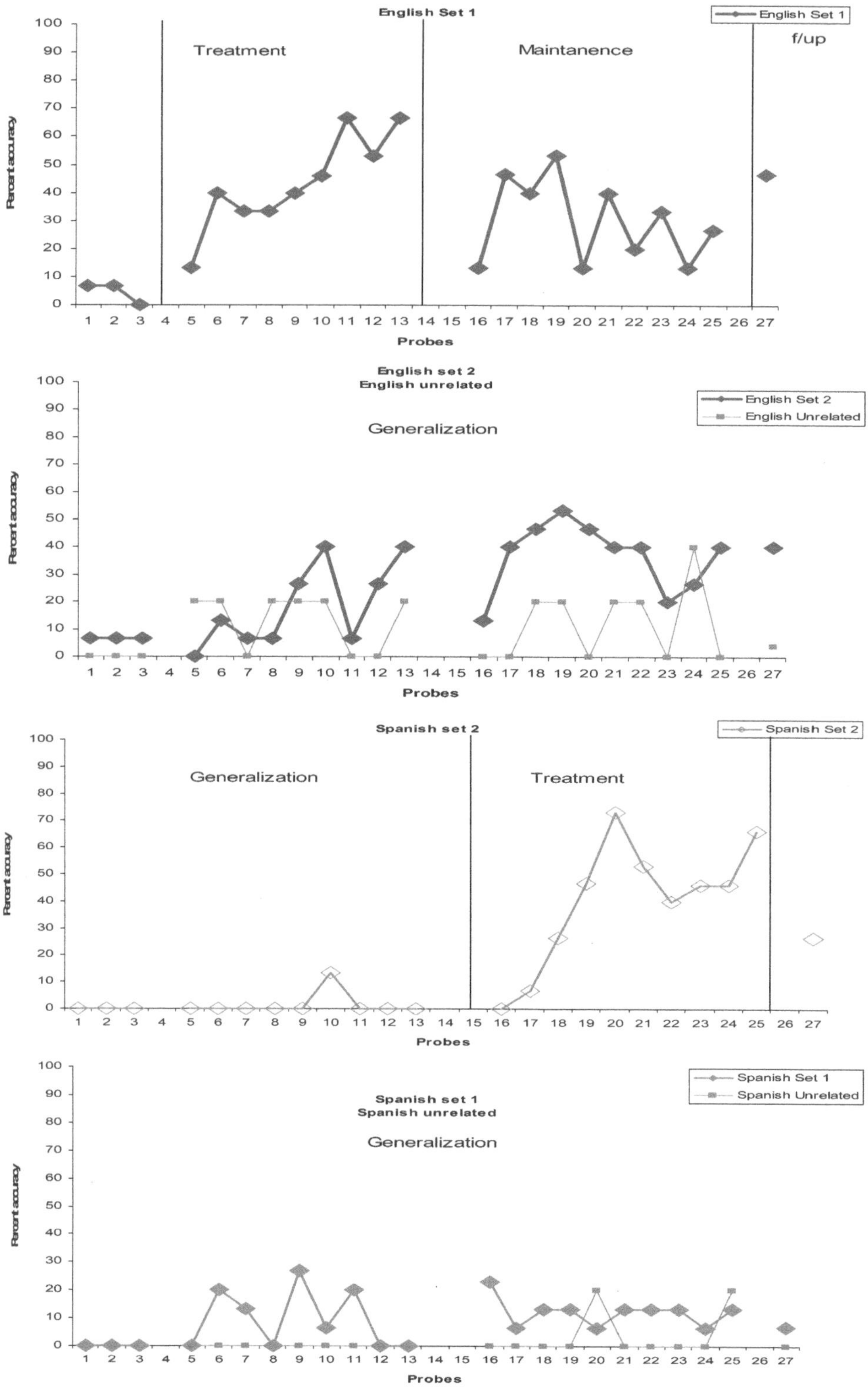

Figure 2. Naming accuracy for Participant 2 on English set 1 (trained first) and English set 2 (semantically related to set 1), and Spanish set 2 (trained second) an Spanish set 1 (translations of English set 1). Control (unrelated) items in English and Spanish are illustrated in the same graph as generalisation items.

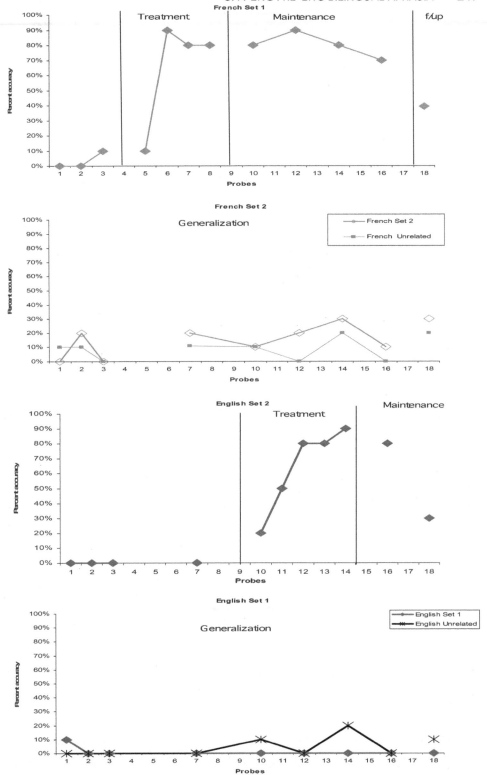

Figure 3. Naming accuracy for Participant 3 on French set 1 (trained first) and French set 2 (semantically related to set 1), and English set 2 (trained second) an English set 1 (translations of English set 1). Control (unrelated) items in English and Spanish are illustrated in the same graph as generalisation items.

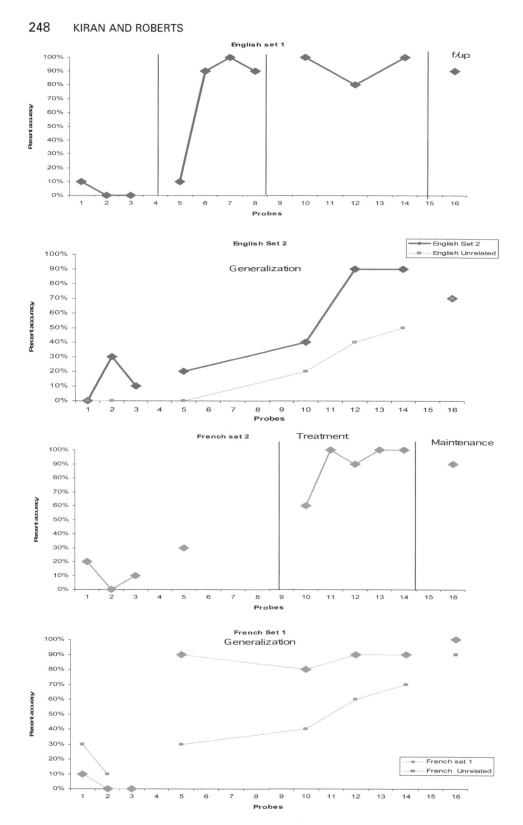

Figure 4. Naming accuracy for Participant 4 on English set 1 (trained first) and English set 2 (semantically related to set 1), and French set 2 (trained second) an French set 1 (translations of English set 1). Control (unrelated) items in English and Spanish are illustrated in the same graph as generalisation items.

Performance improved to a high of 73% but was unstable (ES = 8.8). Surprisingly, performance deteriorated in the semantically related but untrained Spanish words (Spanish set 1) but was overall higher than baseline levels (ES = 2.8). Performance on the untrained English translations of the trained items (i.e., English set 2) showed a variable but ultimately higher average performance (36.6%) than in the previous phase (18.5%) or during baseline (ES = 5.5). Also, performance on the previous trained English set 1 declined slightly (ES = −0.8). Scores for unrelated control items in English (ES = 3.2) and Spanish (ES = 0.5) were unchanged.

Participant 3

P3 was initially trained in French (her stronger language) and then in English. After just one session, naming on the trained items (French set 1) improved dramatically (ES = 13.9). No changes were observed on the untrained but related French set 2 or on the English sets. When treatment shifted to English Set 2, performance on these items jumped to 90% (ES = 11.5), with no change in the semantically related untrained English set 1 (ES = −0.57). Performance on the previously trained French set 1 was maintained after therapy at 70% accuracy for those items that were at 80% when treatment was discontinued. Performance on the untrained French set 2 (ES = 0.98) and the unrelated French control items (ES = 0.26) changed little. Lastly, performance on the unrelated English controls items did not change (ES = 1.03). At follow-up approximately 5 weeks after completing treatment, performance had declined to at or near baseline levels. The patient did not attend two scheduled follow-up appointments to check maintenance/ progress at 3 months post-therapy.

Participant 4

P4 was initially treated in English and then in French. Training on English set 1 resulted in a rapid improvement to a high of 100% (ES = 13.5). Performance at that time on the English semantically related words (set 2) did not change nor did performance on French set 2. However, there was improvement in the French translations of English set 1 (i.e., French set 1) to a high of 90% after treatment in English. Performance on the unrelated English and French items did not change after English treatment.

Treatment was then shifted to French set 2 which improved to a high of 100% in four sessions (ES = 5.8). Performance on the untrained, semantically related French set 1 continued to be highly accurate (ES = 14.5). Her score on the untrained English translations of the trained set (English set 2) improved from 40% to 90% (ES = 3.05). Scores on the unrelated French and English sets improved to a high of 70% (ES = 4.0) and 50% (ES = 2.12) respectively. At follow-up 3 months post-discharge, scores on all sets of words were similar to those at the end of therapy.

Error analysis

For all participants, responses produced during the first baseline session and at the end of treatment for each language (except P1 who only received treatment in Spanish), were coded and are shown in Table 6. P1 showed primarily phonemic and semantic errors in English before Spanish treatment. After treatment in Spanish, the semantic errors remained but there were fewer "no-response" errors. For Spanish stimuli, the main error types were no-responses, neologisms, and semantic errors. After treatment, the main error types were still neologisms, unrelated words, and a few semantic errors.

P2, treated in English then Spanish, showed a variety of errors on English stimuli including no-responses, semantic errors, unrelated words, and neologisms prior to treatment. Even after treatment these error types persisted for the English stimuli. For Spanish stimuli, errors were predominantly no-responses, neologisms, unrelated words, and phonemic errors that were produced before and after treatment. Interestingly, this patient demonstrated more semantic errors in English and more phonemic errors in Spanish. She also showed a tendency to produce semantic errors or the translation of the target in the non-target language.

P3, who was treated first in French then in English, showed predominantly no-responses and semantic errors in English before and after treatment. The pattern was similar for French stimuli: errors were either no-responses or semantic errors prior to treatment. Following treatment, however, semantic errors continued and a few cross-language translations were also observed.

Finally P4, who received treatment first in English and then in French, showed predominantly no responses and semantic errors prior to treatment for both English and French stimuli. Since this patient showed within- and cross-language generalisation, few errors remained post-treatment. These were mainly semantic errors. Interestingly, P3 and P4 made more semantic errors for French stimuli than English stimuli.

Results on standardised tests administered in both languages

Several of the standardised measures that were administered pre-treatment were administered again post-treatment (see Tables 2 and 3). Scores on the *Boston Naming Test* deteriorated in English but improved in Spanish for P1, whereas scores improved in English and Spanish for P2. Slight fluctuations with no specific trends were observed for P3 and P4 (see Figure 5). Performance on the *BAT* fluctuated for the four participants with no apparent pattern.

DISCUSSION

The goals of the present study were to test predictions about bilingual language treatment, and to replicate and extend previous work on cross-language generalisation in bilingual aphasia to new patients and a new language combination (English–French). The experimental design and methodology were very similar to the Edmonds and Kiran (2006) model. Results of the present study revealed somewhat different patterns of results for the four patients. After reviewing the results in light of the five hypotheses proposed in the introduction, we conclude with a discussion of the challenges in conducting and interpreting studies of bilingual aphasia treatment.

Each patient responded differently to the SFA treatment in terms of their improvement on the target items, the within- and between-language generalisation and their maintenance. Table 5 summarises the results and some of the relevant linguistic and other variables for the four patients. For each hypothesis, the results break down as follows:

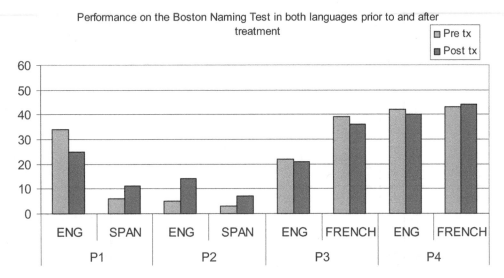

Figure 5. Performance on the Boston Naming Test prior to treatment and after treatment for Participants 1–4. For Participants 1 and 2, performance is shown in English and Spanish and for Participants 3 and 4, performance is shown for English and French.

First, gains on trained items in the trained language occurred for all patients, confirming Hypothesis 1 and providing some support for the efficacy of Semantic Feature Analysis. For P3 and P4, the very rapid improvement and the fact that the trained items improved so much more than the untrained ones strongly suggest that the therapy caused the gains. The improvement may stem from hearing/reading the picture names at least as much as from the strengthened semantic networks in these two patients. However, P1 and P2 failed to reach more than 70% accuracy on the trained words despite the relatively large number of treatment sessions and the fact that they were only 6 months and 11 months post-onset. At least for P1, the lack of robust improvements on the trained items may be influenced by the fact that treatment was provided in her (pre-morbidly) weaker and (post-stroke) more impaired language. Also, both P1 and P2 showed more severe language impairments than P3 and P4.

Second, within-language generalisation occurred for P1, P2, and P4 on items semantically related to the words practiced in therapy, as predicted by Hypothesis 2. However, for P3 this generalisation did not occur.

The cross-language generalisation as predicted by Hypothesis 3 occurred, with clear improvements on translations of the target items for only one of the four patients (P4). Even though P1 showed improvements in English subsequent to treatment in Spanish, the broad improvements of P1 on English set 1 and the increasing scores during the baseline phase make it difficult to interpret her results in terms of this hypothesis. For P2, slight improvements were observed for English set 2 when Spanish set 2 was trained, but again, these results were not robust.

Cross-language generalisation for semantically related targets was predicted by Hypothesis 4, and occurred for P4 and to a lesser extent for P1. While there were improvements in English set 2 for P1, high scores during baseline and the improvement in semantically unrelated words weaken any conclusions drawn from this hypothesis.

TABLE 5
Summary of important pre-stroke language history, post stroke language treatment, and patterns of generalisation observed in the four participants

Participants	P1	P2	P3	P4
MPO	11	6	33	15
Stronger language (self-report)	English	approx equal	French	approx equal
Language of previous tx	English	English	both, more English	almost all English
Language of tx this study (Lt)	Spanish	English, then Spanish	French, then English	English, then French
Number of tx sessions	20 in Spanish	18 in English 20 in Spanish	4 in each language	4 in each language
Reached criterion of ≥80%	No for tx words.	No for all lists in both languages	Yes, in both tx lists	Yes, in both tx lists
Generalisation: within-language	Some, to semantically-related list only	Some during English tx to sem related. Also some, but less, to unrelated words	None	For Eng tx words Eng set 1 to set 2: yes strong.
	Improvement on unrelated words			Some but less to unrelated words during each tx phase
Generalisation: cross-languages	Improvement in English set 2 but questionable	Slight improvement from Spanish set 2 to English set 2	Slight improvement from English set 2 to French set 2	Strong from Eng set 1 (tx) to French set 1; slight to unrelated

MPO: months post onset, tx: treatment, sem: semantic.

TABLE 6
Evolution of errors reported in raw numbers for each patient

	English 1			English 2			English-UNR			Spanish 1			Spanish 2			Spanish-UNR		
	BL	En Tx	Sp Tx	BL	En Tx	Sp Tx	BL	En Tx	Sp Tx	BL	En Tx	Sp Tx	BL	En Tx	Sp Tx	BL	En Tx	Sp Tx
P1	(15)	—	(15)	(15)	—	(15)	(6)	—	(6)	(15)	—	(15)	(15)	—	(15)	(6)	—	(6)
No-Response	1	—	2	2	—	1	3	—	0	5	—	1	3	—	2	3	—	2
Neologism/Perseveration	0	—	0	1	—	0	0	—	0	2	—	5	0	—	0	1	—	3
Unrelated	0	—	1	1	—	1	1	—	0	0	—	1	1	—	3	0	—	1
Phonemic Error-TL	4	—	0	6	—	1	0	—	0	0	—	0	1	—	2	0	—	0
Semantic Error-TL	6	—	4	0	—	2	1	—	1	3	—	1	1	—	2	1	—	0
Circumlocution	0	—	0	0	—	0	0	—	0	0	—	0	0	—	0	0	—	0
Mixed	2	—	0	0	—	0	0	—	0	1	—	0	1	—	0	0	—	0
Phonemic Error-NTL	0	—	0	0	—	1	0	—	0	1	—	0	0	—	0	0	—	0
Semantic Error-NTL	0	—	0	0	—	0	0	—	0	2	—	0	2	—	0	0	—	0
Correct-NTL	0	—	0	0	—	0	1	—	0	1	—	0	2	—	0	1	—	0
Correct-TL	2	—	8	4	—	9	0	—	5	0	—	7	4	—	6	0	—	0
P2	(15)	(15)	(15)	(15)	(15)	(15)	(5)	(5)	(5)	(15)	(15)	(15)	(15)	(15)	(15)	(5)	(5)	(5)
No-Response	7	0	4	5	3	1	0	0	2	3	0	3	9	5	1	0	0	2
Neologism/Perseveration	1	0	1	2	1	1	3	0	0	7	8	6	2	8	1	2	3	2
Unrelated	2	1	1	5	4	2	1	1	1	0	2	3	1	1	0	0	0	0
Phonemic Error-TL	1	4	2	1	2	2	0	0	0	3	5	2	1	0	3	0	1	0
Semantic Error-TL	3	1	3	1	0	2	1	3	1	0	0	0	0	0	0	0	1	0
Circumlocution	0	0	0	0	0	0	0	0	0	0	0	0	0	0	0	0	0	0
Mixed	0	0	0	0	0	0	0	0	0	1	0	0	0	1	0	0	0	0
Phonemic Error-NTL	0	0	0	0	0	1	0	0	0	0	0	0	1	0	0	0	0	0
Semantic Error-NTL	0	0	0	0	0	0	0	0	0	0	0	0	0	0	0	0	0	0
Correct-NTL	0	0	0	0	0	2	0	0	0	1	0	0	1	0	0	2	0	0
Correct -TL	1	9	4	1	5	6	0	1	0	0	0	1	0	0	10	1	0	1

(Continued)

TABLE 6
Continued

	English 1			English 2			English-UNR			French 1			French 2			French-UNR		
	BL	Fr Tx	En Tx	BL	Fr Tx	En Tx	BL	Fr Tx	En Tx	BL	Fr Tx	En Tx	BL	Fr Tx	En Tx	BL	Fr Tx	En Tx
P3	(10)	(10)	(10)	(10)	(10)	(10)	(10)	(10)	(10)	(10)*	(10)	(10)	(10)	(10)	(10)	(10)	(9)	(10)
No-Response	10	9	6	9	8	1	8	6	4	6	2	2	6	3	1	5	2	3
Neologism/Perseveration	0	0	0	0	0	0	0	0	0	0	0	0	0	0	0	0	0	0
Unrelated	0	0	0	0	0	0	0	0	1	0	0	0	1	0	0	0	0	1
Phonemic Error-TL	0	0	0	0	0	0	0	0	0	0	0	0	0	0	0	0	0	0
Semantic Error-TL	0	1	1	1	0	0	2	1	4	3	0	0	3	5	1	2	4	2
Circumlocution	0	0	0	0	0	0	0	2	0	0	0	0	0	0	0	2	3	2
Mixed	0	1	0	0	1	0	0	0	0	0	0	0	0	0	1	0	0	0
Phonemic Error-NTL	0	0	1	0	0	0	0	0	0	0	0	0	0	0	0	0	0	0
Semantic Error-NTL	0	0	0	0	0	0	0	0	0	0	0	0	0	0	0	0	0	0
Correct-NTL	0	0	2	0	0	0	0	0	0	0	0	0	0	2	4	0	0	0
Correct-TL	0	0	0	0	1	9	0	1	1	0	8	8	0	2	3	1	0	2
P4	(10)	(10)	(10)	(10)	(10)	(10)	(10)	(10)	(10)	(10)	(10)	(10)	(10)	(10)	(10)	(10)	(10)	(10)
No-Response	6	0	0	5	0	1	6	0	1	4	0	0	3	0	1	3	0	0
Neologism/Perseveration	0	0	0	1	0	0	0	0	0	1	0	0	0	0	0	0	1	1
Unrelated	0	0	0	1	0	1	0	1	1	0	0	0	0	0	0	1	1	1
Phonemic Error-TL	0	0	0	0	0	0	0	0	0	0	1	1	0	0	0	0	0	0
Semantic Error-TL	4	0	0	2	0	2	2	3	4	3	0	0	3	0	4	3	0	4
Circumlocution	0	0	0	2	0	1	1	1	0	0	0	0	2	0	1	0	1	1
Mixed	0	0	0	0	0	0	1	0	0	1	0	0	0	0	0	0	0	0
Phonemic Error-NTL	0	0	0	0	0	0	0	0	0	0	0	0	0	0	0	0	0	0
Semantic Error-NTL	0	0	0	0	0	0	0	0	2	0	0	0	0	0	0	0	0	0
Correct-NTL	0	0	0	0	0	0	0	0	0	0	0	0	0	0	0	0	0	0
Correct-TL	0	10	10	0	10	4	0	5	2	1	9	9	2	10	4	3	7	4

Numbers in paranthesis indicate the total number of responses for each participant. Please see text for description of error types. TL: Target Language, NTL: Non Target Language; UNR: Unrelated words, **BL**: baseline, SP Tx: probes upon completion of treatment in Spanish, En Tx: probes upon completion of treatment in English, Fr: probes upon completion of treatment in English. * Note that one of the responses in this set was not classifiable.

Finally, as predicted by Hypothesis 5, there was no change in scores for the semantically unrelated words in either language for two patients (P2 and P3). However, for P4 and to a certain extent for P1, the "control words" improved, suggesting that for these patients semantic ties between words were not a critical factor in facilitating improved naming.

Results from the error analysis provide further data regarding each patient's response to treatment. For instance, P4 showed the clearest treatment gains and cross-language generalisation patterns and a predominance of semantic errors. In contrast, P2 never consistently responded to treatment in terms of acquisition and generalisation and showed a variety of errors including neologisms, unrelated words, and phonemic errors that did not change as a function of treatment. P3 showed an increase in correct responses in the non-target language and semantic errors even though she did not demonstrate generalisation. Interestingly, this patient was French dominant pre-morbidly and showed an increase in French responses after English treatment (Correct NTL); but an increase in English responses subsequent to English treatment. Lastly, P1 (English-dominant) showed a decrease in the number of semantic errors in English but not in Spanish even though she received treatment in Spanish.

Both the errors and the generalisation trends are consistent with models referred to in the introduction that posit lexical-semantic connections between L1 and L2 and activation of lexical items in both languages, during work in one language. Specifically, the semantic-based naming treatment improved naming of trained items and semantically related items in the trained language and, in P4 only, to translations in the untrained language. In those cases when naming was incomplete (e.g., P4) errors were predominantly semantic errors or translations in the non-target language. In future studies it would be interesting to see if this error pattern is associated with stronger/easier generalisation. These results, however, are not conclusive in terms of the locus of transfer between the two languages in each patient, so it is impossible to know whether treatment strengthened the direct connections between the translation equivalents in the two languages, and/or indirect connections via the semantic level. This issue should be the focus of future bilingual treatment studies.

Given these limitations, the theoretical conclusions that can be drawn from the present data are tentative. If all four patients had shown similar patterns of results or if the extent and direction of generalisation had varied clearly as a function of the patients' language histories, stronger conclusions would have been possible. However, the current data can only be said to indirectly support the basic tenets of theoretical models proposed by de Groot (1992) and Kroll and Stewart (1994) in as much as they do not contradict them. An important and very positive finding from a clinical standpoint is that the connections are manipulable as a function of treatment.

From a clinical standpoint, these results provide several insights into bilingual aphasia rehabilitation. First, they remind us of how variable the performance of patients can be. As is the case for monolingual patients, some patients respond well to treatment, while other apparently similar patients show little or no improvement (e.g., Laganaro, Di Pietro, & Schnider 2006; Law, Wong, Sung, & Hon, 2006; Marini, Caltagirone, Pasqualetti, & Carlomagno, 2007; Nettleton & Lesser, 1991; Wierenga et al., 2006). After many sessions, P1 and P2 still did not reach 80% correct (12/15), whereas P3 and P4 both jumped to 80% (8/10) or more on their second or third therapy session. Perhaps the relatively mild aphasia of P3 and P4 explains this, and perhaps P2 failed to reach criterion because her aphasia was relatively severe. Also, the larger number of target items for P1 and P2 compared to P3 and P4 may have made it harder to achieve the goal of 80%, although the larger number gives a more representative sample of naming behaviour.

Second, the results remind us that we still do not understand why the performance of only some patients generalises to untrained items. One possible interpretation of the present results is that they replicate and extend those of Edmonds and Kiran (2006). The results for P1 and P4 could even be interpreted as supporting the tentative explanation for the 2006 results; i.e., that treatment in a patient's weaker language is more likely to facilitate generalisation to untrained stimuli than treatment in the patient's stronger language. However, there are other plausible interpretations that cannot be ruled out. The various results for these four patients could be interpreted in terms of their bilingualism (strong/weak languages; age of acquisition of each language; patterns of use). On the other hand, the literature on aphasia treatment in monolingual patients also shows that some patients generalise gains much more than others. So the failure of P3 to generalise from her stronger language to her weaker may have nothing to do with her bilingualism or the stimuli used. Similarly, the generalisation shown by P1 (at 6 months post-onset) may be partly due to spontaneous recovery. Cognitive factors such as executive function have been suggested as a possible explanation for the differing effects of treatment across patients (e.g., Fillingham, Sage, & Lambon Ralph, 2005; Law, Yeung, & Chiu, 2008). Future studies of bilingual patients might be easier to interpret if they include measures of problem solving and other cognitive functions. One way to encourage generalisation is to provide a large number of training sessions (e.g., Raymer, Kohen, & Saffell, 2006) and a larger number of stimuli. Yet after only four sessions in each language, and using only 10 target words, P4 showed strong generalisation within and between languages.

Methodological issues to consider in future studies

The results from the present study raise several issues that cannot be conclusively resolved with the current data and need to be addressed systematically in future studies. For instance, self-reports of proficiency reflect each patient's subjective judgements about their abilities. Although in this study no obvious inconsistencies were found between their language histories, reported age of acquisition, and degree of accentedness in L2, more studies about the validity of self-reports are required. For example, two recent studies showed that participants' self-rated proficiency did not reflect their performance on overt naming (Sebastian & Kiran, 2007) and during semantic priming (Kiran & Lebel, 2007). On the Boston Naming Test, scores correlated modestly with self-rated proficiency in verbal expression at the group level but large variability within each group was found, despite the uniformly high self-ratings of proficiency (Roberts, Garcia, Desrochers, & Hernandez, 2002). There is currently more support for the validity of self-ratings at the group level than for their validity in predicting performance for individuals (see Roberts, 2008, for a review).

A related issue concerns self-reports of age of acquisition for each language. It is difficult to estimate the age of first exposure in older adults. Some do not remember exactly what year English/French/Spanish classes began in school and, even when asked, are unsure about passive exposures through TV, radio, stories; this makes it difficult to reliably classify them and to draw up sets of stimuli that might reflect age of acquisition. It is not clear how important this measure may be for naming recovery, but there is some work suggesting that, especially for priming tasks, and tasks that use reaction time as the dependent variable, there may be word-by-word effects for age of acquisition (e.g., Barry, Johnston, & Wood, 2006; Izura & Ellis, 2002).

One of the difficult aspects of this study was selecting equivalent stimuli in each language. The normal procedure of balancing lists for word length, published word frequency, and for typical age of acquisition is complicated for bilingual speakers. Given Grosjean's (1998) complementarity principle, it is unclear to what extent published word frequency lists for any given language accurately reflect the word frequency or word difficulty for bilingual speakers (Roberts, 2008; Roberts et al., 2002). Even for monolingual speakers, frequency databases that have not separately counted each meaning of homonyms such as *bit* and *mouth* may give very misleading frequency values. Finally, the different samples (written language, Internet, TV shows, newspapers, etc.) used in the word frequency databases and the different ways of calculating frequencies mean that comparing frequencies of a given word in two databases may be invalid.

The validity and reliability of semantic relatedness scores also warrant further study. In the rating exercise, the test–retest reliability was tested by including some pairs more than once, often in reverse order. Mean ratings varied by up to 1 point on a 5-point scale. The extent to which ratings vary with the age and with the level of bilingualism of the raters is unknown. In future studies it would be worthwhile to deliberately vary the degree of relatedness to see if within and/or between language generalisation correlates with rated strength of the semantic ties.

We recognise that the WAB and BNT are not designed to measure aphasia in bilingual speakers. Further, aspects of the BAT require further psychometric scrutiny (e.g., Muñoz & Marquardt, 2008). The ultimate goal of treatment is to effect changes in both languages of bilingual individuals that extend beyond just improvements in naming. Until standardised assessment tools are validated across languages, our ability to make any meaningful interpretations of scores on these tests regarding the severity of aphasia in each language and to measure changes over time in each language is limited.

Conclusion

The present study is the first replication of a bilingual aphasia treatment study across two languages. There are several strengths in the methodology of the study. First, all four participants were relatively similar in age and were all females. The detailed language histories for all patients included comparisons of language use and language history patterns across two pairs of languages. Further, multiple baselines were obtained for all patients and the order of languages treated was counter-balanced across three participants. Consequently the results of the present study allow us to draw some tentative theoretical and clinical conclusions. The present results demonstrate the feasibility of using semantic treatment to facilitate lexical retrieval and generalisation to semantically related untrained items across three different languages. Treatment efficacy was not uniform for all patients, but all patients improved their naming ability. The pattern of improvement in three of the four patients is strongly linked to the phases and targets of the treatment. These results are somewhat equivocal about the extent of transfer to untrained languages, but the treatment has the potential to benefit items in the untrained language. As better methods are developed for selecting stimuli, controlling for more factors related to those stimuli and for grouping patients based on their linguistic histories, a clearer picture will emerge.

REFERENCES

Barry, C., Johnston, R. A., & Wood, R. F. (2006). Effects of age of acquisition, age, and repetition priming on object naming. *Visual Cognition, 13,* 911–927.

Baudot, J. (1992). *Fréquence d'utilisation des mots en français écrit contemporain.* Montréal: Les Presses de l'Université de Montréal.

Beeson, P. M., & Robey, R. R. (2006). Evaluating single-subject treatment research: lessons learned from the aphasia literature. *Neuropsychological Review, 16,* 161–169.

Boyle, M. (2004). Semantic feature analysis treatment for anomia in two fluent aphasia syndromes. *American Journal of Speech-Language Pathology, 13,* 236–249.

Boyle, M., & Coelho, C. (1995). Application of semantic feature analysis as a treatment for aphasic dysnomia. *American Journal of Speech-Language Pathology, 4,* 94–98.

Busk, P. L., & Serlin, R. (1992). Meta analysis for single case research. In T. R. Kratochwill & J. R. Levin (Eds.), *Single case research design and analysis: New directions for psychology and education.* Hillsdale, NJ: Lawrence Erlbaum Associates Inc.

Coelho, C. A., McHugh, R. E., & Boyle, M. (2000). Semantic feature analysis as a treatment for aphasic dysnomia: A replication. *Aphasiology, 14,* 133–142.

Costa, A., & Caramazza, A. (1999). Is lexical selection in bilingual speech production language-specific? Further evidence from Spanish–English and English–Spanish bilinguals. *Bilingualism: Language and Cognition, 2,* 231–244.

Costa, A., La Heij, W., & Navarrete, E. (2006). The dynamics of bilingual lexical access. *Bilingualism: Language and Cognition, 9,* 137–151.

de Groot, A. M. B. (1992). Determinants of word translation. *Journal of Experimental Psychology: Learning, Memory and Cognition, 18,* 1001–1018.

Dijkstra, T., & Van Heuven, W. J. B. (2002). The architecture of the bilingual word recognition system: From identification to decision. *Bilingualism: Language and Cognition, 5,* 175–197.

Drew, R. L., & Thompson, C. K. (1999). Model-based semantic treatment for naming deficits in aphasia. *Journal of Speech, Language, and Hearing Research, 42,* 972–989.

Edmonds, L., & Kiran, S. (2006). Effect of semantic based treatment on cross linguistic generalisation in bilingual aphasia. *Journal of Speech, Language and Hearing Research, 49,* 729–748.

Fillingham, J. K., Sage, K., & Lambon Ralph, M. A. (2005). Further explorations and an overview of errorless and errorful therapy for aphasic word-finding difficulties: The number of naming attempts during therapy affects outcome. *Aphasiology, 19,* 597–614.

Francis, N., & Kucera, H. (1982). *Frequency analysis of English usage.* Boston: Houghton Mifflin.

Green, D. W. (1998). Mental control of the bilingual lexico-semantic system. *Bilingualism: Language and Cognition, 1,* 67–81.

Grosjean, F. (1998). Studying bilinguals: Methodological and conceptual issues. *Bilingualism: Language and Cognition, 1,* 131–149.

Haarbauer-Krupa, J., Moser, L., Smith, G., Sullivan, D., & Szekeres, S. F. (1985). Cognitive rehabilitation therapy: Middle stages of recovery. In M. Ylvisaker (Ed.), *Head injury rehabilitation: Children and adolescents* (pp. 287–310). San Diego, CA: College Hill Press.

Izura, C., & Ellis, C. W. (2002). Age of acquisition effects in word recognition and production in first and second languages. *Psicológica, 23,* 245–281.

Juilland, A., & Chang-Rodriguez, A. (1964). *Frequency dictionary of Spanish words.* London: Mouton & Co.

Kaplan, E., Goodglass, H., & Weintraub, S. (2001). *The Boston Naming Test* (2nd ed.). Baltimore: Lippincott, Williams, & Wilkins.

Kay, J., Lesser, R., & Coltheart, M. (1992). *The Psycholinguistic Assessment of Language Processing in Aphasia (PALPA).* Hove, UK: Lawrence Erlbaum Associates Ltd.

Kertesz, A. (1982). *The Western Aphasia Battery*. Philadelphia: Grune & Stratton.

Kiran, S., & Lebel, K. (2007). Crosslinguistic semantic and translation priming in normal bilingual individuals and bilingual aphasia. *Clinical Linguistics and Phonetics*, *21*, 277.

Kiran, S., & Thompson, C. K. (2003). The role of semantic complexity in treatment of naming deficits: Training semantic categories in fluent aphasia by controlling exemplar typicality. *Journal of Speech, Language, and Hearing Research*, *46*, 773–787.

Kroll, J. F., & Stewart, E. (1994). Category interference in translation and picture naming: Evidence for asymmetric connections between bilingual memory representations. *Journal of Memory and Language*, *33*, 149–174.

Laganaro, M., Di Pietro, M., & Schnider, A. (2006). What does recovery from anomia tell us about the underlying impairment: The case of similar anomic patterns and different recovery. *Neuropsychologia*, *44*, 534–545.

Law, S-P., Wong, W., Sung, F., & Hon, J. (2006). A study of semantic treatment of three Chinese anomic patients. *Neuropsychological Rehabilitation*, *16*, 601–629.

Law, S-P., Yeung, O., & Chiu, K. M. Y. (2008). Treatment for anomia in Chinese using an ortho-phonological cueing method. *Aphasiology*, *22*, 139–163.

Marini, A., Caltagirone, C., Pasqualetti, P., & Carlomagno, S. (2007). Patterns of language improvement in adults with non-chronic, non-fluent aphasia after specific therapies. *Aphasiology*, *21*, 164–186.

Muñoz, M. L., & Marquardt, T. P. (2008). The performance of neurologically normal bilingual speakers of Spanish and English on the short version of the Bilingual Aphasia Test. *Aphasiology*, *22*, 3–19.

Muñoz, M. L., Marquardt, T. P., & Copeland, G. (1999). A comparison of the codeswitching patterns of aphasic and neurologically normal bilingual speakers of English and Spanish. *Brain and Language*, *66*, 249–274.

Nettleton, J., & Lesser, R. (1991). Therapy for naming difficulties in aphasia: Application of a cognitive neuropsychological model. *Journal of Neurolinguistics*, *6*, 139–157.

Paradis, M. (1989). *Bilingual Aphasia Test*. Hillsdale, NJ: Lawrence Erlbaum Associates Inc.

Potter, M., So, K., von Eckardt, B., & Feldman, L. (1984). Lexical and conceptual representation in beginning and proficient bilinguals. *Journal of Verbal Learning and Verbal Behavior*, *23*, 23–38.

Raymer, A. M., Kohen, F. P., & Saffell, D. (2006). Computerised training for impairments of word comprehension and retrieval in aphasia. *Aphasiology*, *20*, 257–268.

Roberts, P. M. (1998). Clinical research needs and issues in bilingual aphasia. *Aphasiology*, *12*, 119–130.

Roberts, P. M. (2008). Issues in assessment and treatment in bilingual and multicultural populations. In R. Chapey (Ed.). *Language intervention strategies in adult aphasia* (5th ed., pp. 245–276). Baltimore: Lippincott, Williams & Wilkins.

Roberts, P. M., & Deslauriers, L. (1999). Picture naming of cognate and non-cognate nouns in bilingual aphasia. *Journal of Communication Disorders*, *32*, 1–23.

Roberts, P. M., Garcia, L. J., Desrochers, A., & Hernandez, D. (2002). English performance of proficient bilingual adults on the Boston Naming Test. *Aphasiology*, *16*, 635–645.

Roberts, P. M., & Kiran, S. (2007). Assessment and treatment of bilingual aphasia and bilingual anomia. In A. Ardila & E. Ramos (Eds.), *Speech and language disorders in bilinguals* (pp. 109–131). New York: Nova Science Publishers.

Roberts, P. M., & Shenker, R. C. (2007). Assessment and treatment of stuttering in bilingual speakers. In R. F. Curlee & E. G. Conture (Eds.), *Stuttering and related disorders of fluency* (3rd ed., pp. 183–210). New York: Thieme Medical Publishers.

Sebastian, R., & Kiran, S. (2007, November). *Semantic processing in Hindi–English bilinguals using fMRI*. Poster, ASHA Convention, Boston, MA.

Silverberg, S., & Samuel, A. G. (2004). The effect of age of second language acquisition on the representation and processing of second language words. *Journal of Memory and Language*, *51*, 381–398.

Wierenga, C. E., Maher, L. M., Moore, A. B., White, K. D., McGregor, K., & Soltysik, D., et al. (2006). Neural substrates of syntactic mapping treatment: An fMRI study of two cases. *Journal of the International Neuropsychological Association*, *12*, 132–146.

APPENDIX

Stimuli and average frequency values (standard deviations in parenthesis) for each patient

English set 1	Spanish set 1	English set 2	Spanish set 2	Average semantic relatedness [1]	English UR	Spanish UR
Participant 1						
Ant	Hormiga	Spider	Arana	1.8	Blanket	Manta
Razor	Rastrillo	Soap	Jabón	2.7	Wallet	Cartera
Leg	Pierna	Arm	Brazo	1.6	Pitcher	Jarra
Cane	Bastón	Umbrella	Paraguas	3.0	Sword	Espada
Sheep	Borrego/ Oveja	Deer	Venado/Ciervo	2.1	Rug	Alfombra
Cloud	Nube	Lightning	Relámpago	2.3		
Eagle	Aguila	Owl	Buho	2.0		
Raccoon	Mapache	Skunk	Zorrillo	2.0		
Shark	Ttiburon	Whale	Ballena	1.7		
Snail	Caracol/ Coconito	Worm	Gusano	2.0		
Nun	Monja	Teacher	Maestra	2.0		
Shelf	Estante	Hook	Gancho	*3.0*		
Stool	Taburete	Counter	Mostrador/ Ventanilla	2.3		
Wheelbarrow	Carretilla	Dustpan	Recogedor	2.3		
Mouth	Boca	Mus-tache	Bigote	2.3		
Participant 2						
Cabbage	Repollo	Radish	Rabano	1.8	Mustache	Tenedor
Dustpan	Recogedor	Vacuum cleaner	Aspiradora	2.0	Garlic	Buho
Forehead	Frente	Chin	Menton	3.0	Deer	Lambriz
Raccoon	Mapache	Skunk	Zorrillo	2.0	Umbrella	Naranja
Razor	Rasador	Soap	Jabon	2.7	Wallet	Meastra
Necklace	Collar	Ring	Anillo			
Shark	Tiburon	Whale	Ballena	1.7		
Counter	Mostrador	Hook	Gancho	2.3		
Stool	Taburette	Shelf	Estante	2.3		
Wheelbarrow	Carretilla	Rake	Rastrillo	2.7		
Newspaper	Periodico	Magazine	*Revista*	1.9		
Robe	Bata	Coat	Abrigo	2.3		
Wrench	Perica	Drill	Taladro	1.6		
Lightning	Relampago	Cloud	*Nube*	*2.3*		
Spider	Arana	Ant	Hormiga	1.8		

English set 1	French set 1	English set 2	French set 2	Average semantic relatedness[2]	English UR	French UR
Participant 3						
Button	Macaron	Badge	Écusson	1.5	Landing	Palier
Ditch	Fossé	Puddle	Flaque	2.3	Cheetah	Guépard
Dragonfly	Libellule	Spider	Araignée	2.3	Clasp	Fermoir
Greenhouse	Serre	Factory	Usine	1.9	Propellers	Hélices
Hinge	Charnière	Bolt	Boulon	2.3	Runway	Piste d'atterisage
Squash	Courge	Eggplant	Aubergine	1.2	Pushpin	Punaise
Stirrups	Étriers	Bit	Mors	1.8	Speaker	Haut parleur
Stopwatch	Chronomètre	Sundial	Cadran solaire	2.5	Helmet	Casque
Swan	Cygne	Partridge	Perdrix	2.1	Wind turbines	Éoliennes
Walrus	Morse	Whale	Baleine	1.6	Spokes	Rayons
Participant 4						
Beetle	Coccinelle	Caterpillar	Chenille	2.4	Carnation	Oeillet
Cuff	Poignet	Tights	Collants	3.0	Firehall	Caserne
Danish	Danoise	Waffle	Gauffre	2.0	Partridge	Perdrix
Fin	Nageoire	Flipper	Palme	1.5	Speaker	Haut parleur
Bit	Mors	Blinders	Oeillères	2.3	Spokes	Rayons
Bolt	Boulon	Hinge	Charnière	2.1	Step ladder	Escabeau
Paperclip	Trombone	Staples	Agraphes	1.4	Clasp	Fermoir
Stopwatch	Chronomètre	Sundial	Cadran solaire	2.4	Landing	Palier
Shingles	Bardeaux	Shutters	Volets	2.5	Starfish	Étoile de mer
Briefcase	Porte-documents	Glasses case	Étui à lunettes	2.2	Button	Macaron

[1]4 point scale; 1 = maximum relatedness. [2]5 point scale; 1 = maximum relatedness.

APHASIOLOGY, 2010, 24 (2), 262–287

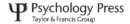
Psychology Press
Taylor & Francis Group

Lexical processing in the bilingual brain: Evidence from grammatical/morphological deficits

Michele Miozzo

University of Cambridge, UK, and Johns Hopkins University, Baltimore, MD, USA

Albert Costa and Mireia Hernández

University of Barcelona, Spain

Brenda Rapp

Johns Hopkins University, Baltimore, MD, USA

Background: A few studies have recently documented cases of proficient bilingual individuals who, subsequent to neural injury, suffered selective deficits affecting specific aspects of lexical processing. These cases involved disruption affecting the production of words from a specific grammatical category (verbs or nouns) or the production of irregular versus regular verb forms. Critically, these selective deficits were manifested in a strikingly similar manner across the two languages spoken by each of the individuals.
Aims: The present study aims at reviewing these cases of selective cross-linguistic deficits and discussing their implications for theories concerning lexical organisation in the bilingual brain.
Methods & Procedures: The studies reviewed here employed a variety of behavioural tests that were specifically designed to investigate the availability in aphasic patients of lexical information concerning nouns and verbs and their morphological characteristics.
Outcomes & Results: The brain-damaged bilingual speakers reviewed in the present study exhibited selective deficits for nouns, verbs, or irregularly inflected verbs in both of their languages.
Conclusions: The selectivity and cross-language nature of the deficits reviewed here indicates that at least certain language substrates are shared in proficient bilingual people. The fact that these deficits affect grammatical class distinctions and verb inflections—information that is part of the lexicon—further indicates that shared neural substrates support lexical processing in proficient bilingual people.

Keywords: Bilingualism; Morphology; Word production; Lexicon.

A significant proportion of the individuals on the planet are proficient bi- or multi-language speakers, able to express themselves with ease in multiple languages,

Address correspondence to: Michele Miozzo, Department of Experimental Psychology, University of Cambridge, Cambridge, CB2 3EB, UK. E-mail: mm584@cam.ac.uk

We wish to thank all of our colleagues who collaborated in the reports we review here. We are especially grateful to Joana Cholin for her essential contributions to the research with WRG. Our recognition also goes to the participants of our studies, for all the efforts they made to allow us an opportunity to understand the nature of their impairments. This research was supported by NIH grants DC006242 (to Michele Miozzo) and DC006740 (to Brenda Rapp) and Spanish Government Grants SEJ-2005/CONSOLIDER-INGENIO (to Albert Costa).

http://www.psypress.com/aphasiology   DOI: 10.1080/02687030902958381

moving from one to the other as the situation demands. How does the brain accomplish such a feat? In an attempt to answer this question researchers have investigated, among other things, how multiple languages are cognitively and neurally organised, how this organisation is similar or different from that of monolingual speakers, and the extent to which this organisation is affected by factors such as level of proficiency or age of acquisition. A wide array of approaches and methodologies have been brought to bear on these questions, including neuroimaging, neuropsychology, and psycholinguistics.

The present paper is a review of the literature specifically concerned with the issue of the production of *words* in multilingual speakers and the extent to which the cognitive and neural substrates of lexical representation and retrieval are shared across languages. We first provide a brief overview of the neuropsychological, neuroimaging, and psycholinguistic literature on the cognitive and neural organisation of multiple languages. Second, we specifically discuss the cognitive architecture of word (lexical) processing in the *monolingual* speaker in order to provide a backdrop for discussion of bilingual lexical processing. Finally, we report on lexical deficits in bilingual aphasia. The focus of this last and major section of the paper is a detailed summary of five neuropsychological case studies that we have previously presented in separate publications (Cholin, Goldberg, Bertz, Rapp, & Miozzo, 2007; de Diego Balaguer, Costa, Sebastián-Gallés, Juncadella, & Caramazza, 2004; Hernández et al., 2008; Hernández, Costa, Sebastián-Gallés, Juncadella, & Reñe, 2007). These case studies concern individuals who exhibit quite selective lexical deficits affecting such things as their ability to orally name words in a particular grammatical category (nouns or verbs) or their ability to produce morphologically irregular vs regular verb forms. Critically, these selective deficits are manifested in a strikingly similar manner across the two languages spoken by the individuals. The cross-language and yet lexically selective nature of the deficits indicates that at least certain language substrates are shared in proficient bilingual people.

THE MULTILINGUAL LANGUAGE SYSTEM: SHARED AND/OR LANGUAGE-SPECIFIC PROCESSES AND SUBSTRATES?

Neuropsychological, neuroimaging, and psycholinguistic research has provided valuable information regarding language representation and processing in the multilingual brain. Each approach has its own logic for drawing conclusions about shared or language-specific structures. In the neuropsychological approach, the observation that an individual exhibits associations/similarities between behavioural deficits across languages is taken as evidence of shared processes and brain structures, while dissociations/differences in abilities across languages indicate independent processes and brain structures. Similarly, with neuroimaging data, overlapping activation patterns produced when participants are processing different languages indicate shared structures, while activation differences indicate at least some degree of independence. Finally, in psycholinguistic research the rationale that has been most commonly employed has considered that evidence that processing in one language either facilitates or interferes with processing in the other language indicates shared structures, while the absence of facilitation or interference suggests independence. In examining the evidence provided by these various approaches, it is important to keep in mind the distinction between shared/independent neural substrates and shared/independent cognitive operations. Psycholinguistic research directly provides information about shared/independent cognitive operations, but only indirectly about their neural substrates. Neuroimaging research operates in a complementary fashion. In either case, however, while shared substrates may certainly imply shared cognitive operations (and vice versa), it is also possible that independent cognitive operations are carried out in common substrates.

An early source of evidence for understanding the brain organisation of language in multilingualism came from the investigations of acquired language deficits in bilingual speakers. Striking among these have been reports of bilingual speakers who have exhibited greater difficulties with one of the languages they had learnt premorbidly or an asymmetry in the pattern of recovery of their language abilities such that one language recovered quickly or more successfully than the other (e.g., Aglioti, Beltramello, Girardi, & Fabbro, 1996; Albert & Obler, 1978; García-Caballero et al., 2007; Gomez-Tortosa, Martin, Gaviria, Charbel, & Ausma, 1995; for reviews see Gollan & Kroll, 2001; Green, 2005; Green & Abutalebi, in press; Paradis, 1977, 2001). At face value, these cross-language differences/dissociations would seem to favour the hypothesis that each language is served by (at least somewhat) independent brain structures. However, the interpretation of this neuropsychological evidence is problematic, as has been pointed out by several investigators. A first difficulty concerns whether language-specific effects could reflect different levels of proficiency and/or use of the two languages, either before or after the neural injury (Green, 2005). The greater familiarity or practice with one language could protect the language from damage or could favour its recovery. In fact, increased exposure to the less-dominant language, *after* the injury, may have facilitated the more rapid recovery of this language relative to the dominant language and may even explain cases of individuals who appear to be less affected in the language that, premorbidly, they had used less frequently or proficiently. Language proficiency and use are often poorly described, making it difficult to establish whether the apparent language-specific impairments actually reflect the neural organisation of the language system or are, instead, the consequence of differential patterns of proficiency and use. Another difficulty in interpreting apparent dissociations has been pointed out by Pitres (1895), Green (1986), and Paradis (1998), and more recently by Abutalebi and collaborators (Abutalebi & Green, 2007; Abutalebi, Miozzo, & Cappa, 2000) who suggested the possibility that dissociations could be the consequence of damage to neural structures that control language switching (most probably subcortical structures like the head of the caudate). Within this interpretation, selective impairment to one language can be explained as a failure of the switching mechanism, a situation that can render one language largely or sporadically unavailable. This type of explanation does not require positing independent brain structures dedicated to each language.[1]

With regard to neuroimaging evidence, a number of researchers have concurred that a general picture is emerging from the body of neuroimaging research on bilingualism, despite the variety of tasks, languages, and bilingual groups examined in these studies (Abutalebi, Cappa, & Perani, 2001; Abutalebi & Green, 2007;

---

[1] It is also likely that researchers have a bias for reporting multilingual aphasic individuals who exhibit discrepancies—of one sort or another—between the two languages. This may be because they are concerned that results showing similarly impaired languages may be ambiguous in their interpretation. Such a bias may prevent us from obtaining data that would bolster the plausibility of shared brain structures.

Indefrey, 2006; Stowe & Sabouring, 2005). The neuroimaging data, however, generally point to a different conclusion from the neuropsychological data. Most of the neuroimaging studies have shown fairly comparable levels of activation in overlapping brain structures when relatively proficient bilingual people performed language tasks in each of their languages. Moreover, these overlapping structures have tended to coincide with the left hemisphere areas that are activated when monolingual speakers produce or read words (e.g., Chee, Hon, Lee, & Soon, 2001; Chee, Soon, Lee, Pallier, 2004; Hernandez, Dapretto, Mazziotta, Bookheimer, 2001; Klein, Watkins, Zatorre, & Milner, 2006; Wartenburger et al., 2003). Differences in the distribution of brain activation between the two languages have been typically reported for bilingual people who were not very proficient or had just started second language acquisition, and these differences have typically taken the form of greater extension of the activated area for the second language (L2). This finding has been attributed to a variety of causes, including the need for greater suppression of the first language (L1) when using L2 (Green, Crinion & Price, 2006) or the involvement of larger neuronal population in relatively novel tasks/skills (Indefrey, 2006), a result that is reported in a number of domains. Overall, the neuroimaging data lend some support to the idea that common brain structures are involved in processing both of the languages spoken by proficient bilingual people. However, the characteristics of current neuroimaging techniques and approaches also require caution in drawing firm conclusions. The fact that shared activation across languages was observed in aggregated data obtained from groups of participants may have obscured L1–L2 differences present at individual level, or may have prevented detection of activation differences that were rather small or involved relatively small brain areas. Furthermore, although most of the results with proficient bilingual people have indicated activation in overlapping areas, there are also several results that have reported language-specific activation (e.g., Dehaene et al., 1997; Kovelman, Baker, & Petitto, 2008; Perani et al., 2003; Wartenburger et al., 2003).

Stimulation of cortex with a briefly presented electrical current while an individual is fully conscious allows for short-lived, transient disruptions of cognitive operations. This procedure is most often carried out for the purposes of mapping the substrates of critical cognitive functions in individuals prior to surgical resection of tumours or epileptic foci (Ojemann, 1995) and may provide a powerful means of addressing question regarding shared/independent substrates of multilingual language processing. For example, electrical stimulation data reported by Lucas, McKhann, and Ojemann (2004) suggest that both shared and language-specific areas co-exist in proficient bilingual people. Lucas et al. (2004) used this technique to identify areas involved in object naming in L1 and L2. In almost all the participants it was possible to isolate areas in which electrical stimulation disrupted naming in both languages (shared areas), and areas in which naming was impaired in only one language (language-specific areas). Both shared and language-specific areas were located in the left perisylvian regions that are also pivotal for language processing in monolinguals. While the results from electrical stimulation may be seen as adding complexity to the issue of language organisation in bilingual brains, they also raise the possibility that the seemingly discrepant findings from neuropsychology and neuroimaging may be a consequence of the different propensities of these techniques—the former for uncovering language-specific areas, the latter for identifying shared areas, with the truth being that both exist.

The co-existence of shared and language-specific areas is in line with psycholinguistic research and the proposals about bilingual processing that have been developed based on this work. These proposals typically draw a distinction between processes and representations that are shared across languages and those that are language-specific. Several proposals concur that semantic processes are, for the most part, shared across languages (e.g., Costa, Miozzo, & Caramazza, 1999; Hermans, Bongaerts, De Bot, & Scheuder, 1998; Kirsner, Smith, Lockhart, King, & Jain, 1984; Kroll & Stewart, 1994; La Heij et al., 1990; Potter, Von Eckardt, & Feldman, 1984; for a review, see Kroll & Tokowicz, 2005; Malt, Sloman, Gennari, Shi, & Wang, 1999). Within such proposals, language specificity is typically limited to syntactic and lexical processes, which may be a consequence of the fact that languages differ more in their lexical and syntactic properties than their semantic ones. Furthermore, it may be that computational segregation of lexical and syntactic processing is required for efficiency. For example, Costa et al. (1999) hypothesised that the efficient word production demonstrated by proficient bilingual speakers relies on computationally separating the two lexicons and restricting lexical access to the language selected for speaking. This lexical segregation may be accomplished through suppression of the non-target language (e.g., Green, 1998). How this segregation is instantiated neurally is not addressed by the psycholinguistic work. Segregation may involve separate neural substrates for the different languages, or a common neural network that can be differentially accessed with inhibitory mechanisms playing an important role. Despite the arguments favouring language specificity in lexical and syntactic processes and representation, there is also considerable psycholinguistic evidence that languages may interact in the course of lexical retrieval. Evidence for this comes from research on cognates—words with the same meaning and same or similar form across languages, for example *pear* and its Spanish equivalent *pera*. Various lines of evidence have demonstrated that cognates can be produced more quickly and with fewer errors than non-cognates matched for variables affecting word production (Costa, Caramazza, & Sebastián-Gallés, 2000; Gollan & Acenas, 2004). Although not the only explanation, the facilitatory effects of cognates can be readily explained if it is assumed that the words of both languages are activated—the convergence of activation on identical word sounds makes word production easier (see Costa, Santestban, & Caño, 2005).

Finally, it is worth recalling that quite possibly the most significant insight of modern theoretical linguistics has been the understanding that beneath the many differences one can observe across languages, there is a common underlying grammatical structure in each of the linguistic domains—from phonetics and phonology, to morphology and syntax (Greenberg, 1976). This common, underlying fabric of languages makes it plausible that the same neural substrates that support language processing in different speakers of different languages also support the different languages that speakers of multiple languages acquired early in their lives. Therefore, research in theoretical linguistics adds plausibility to the hypothesis that even syntactic and lexical mechanisms, which vary so extensively cross-linguistically, could be subserved by common substrates (at least in speakers who acquired multiple languages at an early age).

The evidence we have reviewed up to this point makes it evident that current empirical results do not allow a confident answer to the question of whether shared and/or language-specific neural substrates support language processing in proficient bilingual speakers. That is, even if evidence from neuroimaging and electrical stimulation is correct in indicating that at least some substrates are shared, fundamental uncertainties remain about the particular cognitive functions associated with these areas. In the next section we provide a brief overview of the architecture of lexical processing and representation that may be assumed to be in place in the monolingual speaker. Then, with this foundation, in the main section of the paper we go on to consider the neuropsychological data from aphasic bilingual speakers who suffer from deficits that specifically affect the retrieval and processing of word forms.

THE MULTI-COMPONENT LEXICAL SYSTEM OF THE MONOLINGUAL SPEAKER

The term *lexical* refers to the multiple aspects of our knowledge of words: the semantic, syntactic, and form (phonological and orthographic) properties of each word that is familiar to a speaker. For example, the lexical information corresponding to the English word *cat* would include reference to its meaning (the semantic features characterising at least the defining aspects of the concept, such as "feline", "pet", "furry"), its syntactic features (noun, countable), a specification of its morphological properties (it takes the regular -*s* inflection in the plural), a complete list of its phonological features (its constituent phonemes and their positions, the syllable structure of the word and its stress pattern), as well as information regarding the letters that make up the spelling of the word. All of this information is relevant for word production prior to engaging the motor and pre-motor systems.

In the monolingual speaker there is considerable evidence that these various aspects of lexical knowledge are represented and stored with sufficient independence that brain injury may disrupt one aspect of lexical processing while sparing others (see Rapp & Goldrick, 2006, for a review). The independence of lexical-semantic information from other aspects of lexical knowledge finds support from two lines of evidence: neuropsychological results, which demonstrate highly selective deficits for semantic vs other lexical knowledge (for a review of this evidence see Hillis, 2001), and neuroimaging findings, which show that distinct neural circuitries are associated with semantic and other lexical features (e.g., Miceli et al., 2002). With regard to grammatical information, there is also evidence from aphasia indicating that grammatical information associated with a word may be available when the phonological and orthographic forms of the word are not. For example, Miozzo and collaborators reported on individuals who could indicate specific grammatical properties of Italian nouns (gender) and verbs (the type of the associated auxiliary verb) even when they could not produce the name or answer questions about the sounds in the word (Badecker, Miozzo, & Zanuttini, 1997; Miozzo & Caramazza, 1997). Finally, there are numerous results indicating that knowledge of the orthographic and phonological forms of words may be selectively affected by neural injury leaving intact semantic and syntactic knowledge, this is particularly evident in cases of anomia (e.g., Kay & Ellis, 1987; Lambon-Ralph, Sage, & Roberts, 2000).

In addition to the overall "tripartite" componential organisation of the lexical system that distinguishes between semantic, grammatical, and form knowledge, there are a number of results that reveal the internal complexity of these individual components. In this paper our focus will be on the internal organisation and content of what we will refer to as "the word-form system" responsible for the storage, retrieval, and processing of phonological and orthographic word forms, with major subcomponents sometimes referred to as the phonological and orthographic lexicons. Research has provided evidence that the word-form system is internally complex.

First, there is evidence that orthographic and phonological word forms can be independently represented and processed, a claim supported by the striking cases of individuals who can write the forms of words that they cannot say and vice versa (see Rapp & Goldrick, 2006). In addition, there is evidence that the word-form system is organised in a manner that distinguishes between grammatical categories (nouns/verbs/closed class). The evidence for this comes from individuals who exhibit selective difficulties in naming words of one grammatical category, revealing that word forms corresponding to the different grammatical categories are stored and/or retrieved with at least some neural independence from one another.[2] Converging evidence has also come for neuroimaging where there have been successful attempts to segregate effects of grammatical class from effects of concreteness or other semantic variables (Berlingeri et al., 2008). In addition to knowledge of a word's grammatical category, the word-form component includes information and procedures that allow for the morphological changes (changes in word form) that a word can undergo. For example, in English, a noun's lexical representation includes information and procedures that allow for the proper formation of the plural. For most nouns, this is accomplished with the addition of an -s to the stem, but there is also the idiosyncratic or "irregular" plural formation seen in words such as *goose* → *geese*, *man* → *men*, and *sheep* → *sheep*. Similarly, with English verbs, information and procedures allow for the inflectional processes that produce tense and number/person. As is the case for English nouns, we find that while the majority of English verbs follow a "regular" and predictable pattern of inflection (-*ed*) in the past tense, there are a considerable number that do not, and are referred to as irregular (*go* → *went*, *buy* → *bought*, *hit* → *hit*). The lexicon must represent the information and procedures necessary to achieve the fluent generation of these forms, and psycholinguistic studies have demonstrated that the distinction between regular and irregular inflections has also consequences for word processing and lexical acquisition (for a review, see Marcus, 2000; Ullman 2001). Similarly, analyses of language impairments, both developmental and acquired, have demonstrated that regular and irregular inflectional processes can be selectively impaired (e.g., Cortese, Balota, Sergent-Marshall, Buckner, & Gold, 2006; Miozzo, 2003; Miozzo & Gordon, 2005; Patterson, Lambon-Ralph, Hodges, & McClelland, 2001; Penke, Janssen, & Krause, 1999; Tyler, Randall, & Marslen-Wilson, 2002; Ullman et al., 1997; Ullman & Gopnik, 1999).

Questions regarding the processing of regular and irregular inflections have provoked highly contentious debates; nonetheless, current accounts converge in proposing that the regular/irregular distinction has a neurocognitive basis. That is, distinct brain mechanisms are assumed to support the processing of regular and irregular inflections. One way of conceptualising the distinction between regular and

---

[2] One concern has been that these dissociations could reflect the neural organisation of areas devoted to semantic knowledge, within which objects and actions could be distinctly represented (e.g., as a result of differential interactions with motor/object recognition areas). However, in at least some cases it has been shown that the grammatical class deficits can occur in the context of preserved semantic processing (Shapiro, Shelton, & Caramazza, 2000; Zingeser & Berndt, 1988) and, moreover, selective deficits for nouns or verbs have been shown to occur in only one output modality (either spoken or written; Caramazza & Hillis, 1991; Rapp & Caramazza, 1998). Thus, the neuropsychological data demonstrate that deficits for nouns and verbs cannot always be reduced to semantic deficits and point instead to a distinction between nouns and verbs that is present at the level of word form retrieval/representation.

irregular inflection in English assumes that the storage and retrieval of lexical material plays a critical role for irregular forms (Pinker, 1991; Ullman et al., 1997). Specifically, it has been proposed that irregularly inflected forms (e.g., *men, geese, oxen; went, fought, dug*) are stored (memorised) and retrieved as whole words from memory, whereas regularly inflected forms (e.g., *cats, bananas; walked; remembered*) are generated by combining stems (*cat* or *walk*) and the default inflections (*-s, -ed*) (but see Joanisse & Seidenberg, 1999, and Rumelhart & McClelland, 1986, for alternative proposals). Given these assumptions, it is clear that the efficient storage and retrieval of morphological elements (stems, affixes, irregular forms) are critical for morphological operations. As a result, we would expect individuals with difficulties in lexical retrieval to have morphological difficulties and we would expect especial difficulties with the irregular forms of nouns and/or verbs (e.g., *geese, bought*), as these are particularly reliant on lexical retrieval.

In sum, producing a written or spoken word requires the recruitment and coordination of the various components and operations of the lexical system, including: specifying the meaning of the word to be produced, recovering its grammatical features, retrieving its phonological and/or orthographic form, and engaging the requisite morphological processes. In the context of the multilingual brain, one can ask: To what extent are these various lexical processes shared or independent across a speaker's languages? Just as patterns of impaired and spared performance have shed considerable light on the nature of the lexical system in monolingual speakers, we can expect that the study of bi- and multilingual speakers will constitute an equally rich source of information. In the next section we review cases in the literature that provide information relevant to the question of the organisation of the multilingual lexical processing system, focusing on five individuals we have reported in previous work.

MULTILINGUAL LEXICAL RETRIEVAL: EVIDENCE FROM APHASIA

There are few reports in the bilingual aphasia literature that can be clearly identified as specifically involving lexical retrieval deficits; that is, deficits that affect the retrieval and processing of word forms. A key component in establishing lexical retrieval failure is showing that the other processes involved in word production are either intact or not responsible for the critical word production impairment. Critically, both semantic and articulatory or motoric (post-lexical) deficits must be ruled out as the source of the pattern of interest. Therefore, although there may be a number of cases of lexical retrieval deficits in the bilingual aphasia literature, sufficient information is not always provided to allow for a clear localisation of the deficit. We organise our summary below into two sections, the first dealing with grammatical category deficits, the second dealing with lexical retrieval deficits that specifically result in greater accuracy in the production of regular vs irregular verb forms. As the review will show, these cases all involve highly similar deficits in both languages, providing support for the hypothesis that at least some aspects of lexical representation and retrieval are shared across languages.

Grammatical category impairments in bilingual aphasia

As indicated earlier, evidence from monolingual speakers has revealed that word-forms of different grammatical categories are organised with sufficient independence from one another such that retrieval of words in one grammatical category can be selectively disrupted. The cases described in this section indicate that this category-specific organisation may be instantiated in neural substrates that are shared across languages in bilingual speakers.

One relevant report is that of Almagro, Sanchez-Casas, and Garcia-Albea (2003) in which a Catalan–Spanish aphasic speaker is described as having greater difficulties in orally producing nouns than verbs in both languages (although the deficit was more severe in Catalan, L1). A semantic locus was unlikely as this individual exhibited good performance in word–picture matching. Although he did appear to have some (post-lexical) articulatory difficulty, this should not have affected nouns more than verbs, and therefore is unlikely to have been the source of the grammatical category dissociation. The finding of such a selective deficit that affects multiple languages clearly provides support for a shared-substrates view of bilingual lexical representation. Two other cases similar to the Almagro et al. (2003) case, and for which we have somewhat more detailed information have been reported by Hernández, et al. (2007, 2008).

Like the Almagro et al. (2003) case, both of the Hernandez et al. cases involved Spanish–Catalan bilinguals. Nouns and verbs exhibit similar morphological characteristics in Catalan and Spanish. In both languages, nouns are marked for grammatical gender and number, while their verbs carry inflections denoting tense, person, and number and are organised within similar conjugational systems. These morphological similarities make the two languages more comparable, facilitating a comparison between them. The inflections taken by the nouns and verbs in the two languages can either be the same (e.g., -a for singular, feminine nouns; -é for the future tense, first person of verbs) or different (e.g., the suffix –c is used with present tense, first person singular verbs in Catalan but not in Spanish). Similarities between Catalan and Spanish are also evident at the word-form level with many verb and noun cognates (e.g., *porta/puerta* [door], *ballar/bailar* [to dance]). However, the high number of Catalan/Spanish cognates complicates the comparison of responses in the two languages. Cognates may allow for apparently correct responses in both languages, even if responses were available in only one language. To circumvent this problem, results should be confirmed with words that are unique in each language.

Both individuals described by Hernandez et al. (2007, 2008) exhibited word-finding difficulties as a result of degenerative neuropathologies (see the Appendix for more detailed case history information). LPM was diagnosed with a possible dementia of Alzheimer type (AD), and primary progressive aphasia (PPA) was suspected for patient JPG. JPG's suffered a relatively rapid decline of language skills, which were monitored by testing him at regular intervals for 18 months. Before the onset of their illnesses, both individuals were fluent in Catalan and Spanish, languages that they had spoken regularly during their daily activities. Both individuals first acquired one language—Catalan for LPM, Spanish for JPG—but were exposed to both languages early in life.

The same picture set was administered to both individuals, thus allowing a direct comparison of their contrasting performance. The set consisted of an equal number of pictures ($N = 36$) showing objects and actions, which had been selected to elicit nouns and verbs, respectively (see Hernández et al., 2007 for details on the materials). Participants were instructed to name the actions using verbs inflected in the present participle. Nouns and verbs were matched for (lemma) frequency and length (number of phonemes), both in Catalan and Spanish. Nouns and verbs were also comparable with respect to concreteness and imageability, variables that prior research has demonstrated may be responsible for asymmetries in noun/verb naming (Bird, Howard, & Franklin, 2000; Marshall, Chiat, Robson, & Pring, 1996a; Marshall, Pring, Chiat, & Robson, 1996b). Similar numbers of Spanish–Catalan cognates were included within each list (33/36 cognates among nouns and 26/36 cognates among verbs). When administered to a control group of AD patients, nouns and verbs were named equally successfully in Spanish (Hernández et al., 2007), a result demonstrating that the materials employed to elicit nouns and verbs were well equated in terms of difficulty.

The results of oral picture naming revealed that LPM and JPG showed a different performance pattern than the controls in both of the languages in which they were tested. LPM named nouns significantly less accurately than verbs in L1, Catalan (39% vs 78%; $\chi^2 = 9.57$, $p = .002$), as well as in L2, Spanish (28% vs 67%; $\chi^2 = 10.92$, $p = .001$). A more dramatic illustration of LPM's noun-naming difficulties came from a second list of pictures shown only to LPM. Each picture depicted an action that involved an object (e.g., hammering). LPM was asked to name the action and the object—he was more likely to succeed with the former (76% correct) than the latter (36% correct; $\chi^2 = 8.93$, $p = .003$). Circumlocutions accounted for most of LPM's errors in Catalan (71%) and in Spanish (60%).

In contrast, JPG's naming difficulties were significantly more severe for verbs than nouns, although his naming performance varied over time and between languages, as illustrated in Figure 1. During the first year of testing, JPG's naming of nouns in L1 (Spanish) remained relatively accurate (about 80% correct); during this time, his naming of verbs in L1 declined steadily (dropping from 58% to 35%). When the results are collapsed across the four testing sessions of the first year, accuracy was 84% for nouns and 44% for verbs ($\chi^2 = 98.52$, $p = .0001$). Towards the end of the investigation, JPG's naming in L1 deteriorated severely even for nouns, which came to be named as poorly as verbs. Naming in L2 (Catalan) was less accurate and subject to a faster decline than naming in L1. Thus, accuracy was lower in L2 than L1, and a significant difference between nouns and verbs was observed in L2 only within the first 6 months of testing (accuracy, nouns = 31%; verbs = 15%; $\chi^2 = 9.51$, $p = .002$). Further evidence suggesting a relatively more severe impairment for L2 comes from JPG's errors. On a significant proportion of trials (70/288, 24%), JPG responded in Spanish when a response was expected in Catalan. However, he rarely gave a response in Catalan while attempting to name pictures in Spanish (3/147, 2%). Overall, omissions (don't know responses) represented the most common type of error produced by JPG in L1 (71%) as well as in L2 (67%). Because contrasting grammatical class effects were observed in LPM and JPG with the same materials in the same task, we can rule out stimulus confounds as a possible explanation of their selective deficits for nouns and verbs.[3]

As we mentioned above, cognates are common between Catalan and Spanish and represent another variable one should control carefully. Recent data, obtained with normal speakers, have shown that cognates are less susceptible to errors (Gollan & Acenas, 2004), can be named more quickly (e.g., Costa et al., 2000), and require less brain activation in non-proficient bilingual speakers (De Bleser et al., 2003). Of more

---

[3] Selective difficulties with either nouns or verbs have also been documented in monolingual individuals with AD or other forms of dementias (e.g., Hillis, Tuffiash, & Caramazza, 2002; Parris & Weekes, 2001; Robinson, Grossman, White-Devine, & D'Esposito, 1996).

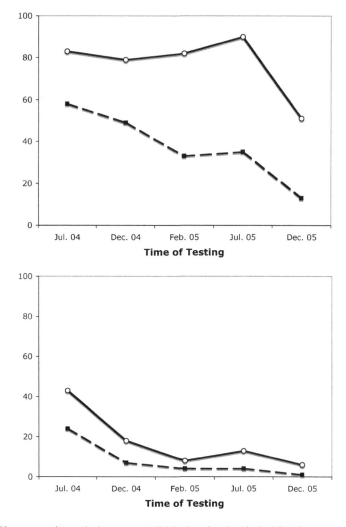

Figure 1. JPG's accuracy in producing nouns (solid line) and verbs (dashed line) in response to pictures of objects and actions, respectively. Responses obtained in oral naming at different testing times in L1 (Spanish) (top graph) and L2 (Catalan) (bottom graph).

direct relevance in the present context, it has also been reported that bilingual aphasic people are more accurate in naming pictures with cognate nouns than non-cognate nouns (Roberts & Deslauriers, 1999). To the extent that cognates may also be protected from brain damage or require less activation, it is important to determine if cognates contributed to a patient's correct responses. A control of cognates is especially important when similar results are obtained across languages— as is the case with LPM and JPG. With cognates, accessing one language might be sufficient to guess or prime the responses in the other language, creating the impression that both languages are equally accessible when in fact they are not. The cognate effect was assessed with LPM using a set of pictures consisting of an equal number of cognate and non-cognate nouns and verbs. This list also produced a grammatical class effect (% correct, nouns vs verbs: L1 = 24% vs. 67%, L2 = 24% vs 54%), but what is crucial is that the accuracy of LPM's responses did not differ significantly between cognates and non-cognates in L1 (65% vs 54%) and L2 (48% vs 27%). This result rules out that the cognate status of the words accounts for LPM's similar performance across languages. The same conclusion holds for JPG, although the cognate effect could be tested less systematically and only through a post-hoc analysis of his picture naming responses. Most of the pictures named by JPG were Spanish/Catalan cognates, but of two types. Some pictures had identical names in Spanish and Catalan—an example is *cow*, which is *"vaca"* in both languages. Other pictures had names that differed slightly in the two languages—an example is *heart*, which is *corazón* in Spanish and *cor* in Catalan. In both languages, JPG's responses were significantly less accurate for verbs than nouns for both identical and non-identical cognates (χ^2s with $p < .01$).

As discussed earlier in this paper (see Footnote 2), selective deficits for nouns and verbs can sometimes be explained in terms of semantic-level failures to identify objects or actions. This possibility is of potential concern since in the materials used in testing LPM and JPG, the noun/verb distinction and the object/action distinction were conflated. Furthermore, to the extent that semantic representations support naming in both languages, a semantic deficit affecting either the category of actions or objects would be expected to occur across languages. However, with LPM there are two results that are not consistent with a semantic interpretation of his selective noun deficit. First, in a comprehension task LPM was quite successful both with verbs (93% correct) and with nouns (95% correct) in matching a spoken word to its corresponding picture among two picture distractors that were semantically related to the target. Second, LPM's errors in oral naming were rarely semantically related to the target (9/68, 13%; data collapsed between L1 and L2), unlike what has been reported in patients with naming impairments arising from a disruption at the semantic level. On this basis we can be fairly confident that the selective difficulty that LPM experienced in naming nouns arose at a post-semantic level of word retrieval. The picture with JPG is a bit more complex. Like LPM, JPG also made very few semantic errors in the verbal picture-naming task (37/435 errors, 8%; data collapsed across languages and testing sessions). However, in the word–picture matching task with semantically related foils, JPG had greater difficulties with verbs than nouns. For example, in one of the initial testing sessions, JPG's responded significantly more accurately to nouns than verbs in L1 (97% vs 75%; $\chi^2 = 5.69$, $p = .01$)—although not in L2 (nouns = 92%, verbs = 83%; *ns*). Nonetheless, if the difficulties that JPG experienced with verbs in naming and comprehension originated entirely from a semantic deficit, then one might expect (a) for JPG to perform similarly in the two tasks and (b) for both languages to be similarly affected. However, while in picture naming L1 and L2 showed a similar dissociation with verbs better than nouns, in the word–picture matching task there was never a statistically significant dissociation between the two categories. Furthermore, while in picture naming JPG's accuracy declined over time with verbs in L1 (from 58% to 35% correct), his performance in L1 did not decline over the same time period in the word-picture matching task that indexes semantic integrity (75% to 72%). These results make it unlikely that a semantic impairment can fully explain JPG's selective verb naming deficit across the two languages.

In sum, the double dissociation of noun and verb naming observed in LPM and JPG is most likely due to a disruption in accessing information regarding the phonological forms of nouns or verbs. Importantly, the specificity of the pattern and the fact that it occurred across languages, indicates that the grammatical category organisation of word-form knowledge observed in monolingual speakers is also present in proficient bilingual speakers and is likely to be based on shared cognitive and neural mechanisms.

Deficits in the production of irregularly inflected forms in bilingual aphasia

In this section we review the cases of bilingual aphasia in which a selective difficulty with irregularly inflected forms has been reported. Given the architecture for monolingual word production reviewed above, such deficits should originate in the retrieval of word-forms or stems and/or in the retrieval of the specific morphological information required to correctly carry out verb inflection. We describe two cases reported by de Diego Balaguer et al. (2004) and one reported by Cholin et al. (2007).

The first two cases of bilingual individuals with aphasia exhibiting selective difficulty in producing irregular forms in both of their languages—Spanish and Catalan—were reported by de Diego Balaguer et al. (2004). In Spanish and Catalan, most verbs have predictable inflections, with the exception of a number of irregular verbs, which take forms deviating from this regular pattern. As in English, the regular/irregular status of verbs does not reliably correlate with their semantics or phonology—it is a rather idiosyncratic and unpredictable feature. The verb systems in Spanish and Catalan are relatively complex, in part because verbs have a fairly large number of tenses, each marked by different inflections, although verbs do cluster into three families (conjugations), which differ with regard to their inflections. Here it suffices to highlight certain features that are common to the verb systems of both languages (for further details about Spanish and Catalan verbs, see de Diego Balaguer et al., 2004). It is important to note that regular and irregular verbs take the same inflections marking person, number, and tense—what makes verbs irregular are variations in the stem. For example, the irregular Spanish verb *pedir* [to ask] takes the stems *ped-* and *pid-*, while the Spanish verb *salir* [to exit] has the stems *sal-* and *salg-*. Furthermore, the tense with which the irregular stems are associated may vary across verbs. For example, for *pedir*, the irregular stem *pid-* surfaces with the three singular forms as well as with the third person plural form. With *salir*, however, the irregular stem *salg-* appears only with the first person singular. It should also be emphasised that whether a verb is regular or irregular varies widely between Catalan and Spanish, so that verbs that are regular in one language may be irregular in the other language. This even holds also for cognate verbs—verbs with phonologically similar forms in Spanish and Catalan; for example, *sento* ([I] feel) is regular in Catalan while its Spanish translation *siento* is irregular. Moreover, the inflectional material itself differs between the two languages (e.g., the verb suffix *-c* is found in Catalan but not in Spanish). Given this high degree of unpredictability, it is natural to assume that information regarding which specific verbs take irregular stems for which specific tenses must be stored in the lexical system, as well as the particular phonological forms taken by these verbs. It would not be surprising, therefore, that deficits affecting lexical retrieval should have a special impact on the production of irregular verb forms.

De Diego Balaguer et al. (2004) reported two individuals—JM and MP—both of whom spoke Spanish and Catalan fluently and on a regular basis before the strokes that left them aphasic. Each of these individuals acquired one language first: Spanish for JM, Catalan for MP, and the other language at an early age. Subsequent to their strokes both individuals exhibited word-naming difficulties in spontaneous speech and in picture naming. JM was 73% and 78% correct in picture naming in Spanish and Catalan respectively, with errors consisting primarily of circumlocutions, omissions or morphological errors. Similarly, MP was 78% and 72% correct in Catalan and Spanish respectively, with errors also consisting primarily of circumlocutions and omissions. A semantic locus of impairment was an unlikely source of these errors, as both individuals performed with high accuracy in both languages on several spoken and written word-picture matching tasks with semantic distractors (JM: 100% correct; MP: 83–100% correct).

Given the lexical retrieval deficits exhibited by both of these individuals in both languages, their spoken production of regularly and irregularly inflected verbs is of particular interest. Both individuals were tested using a sentence completion task that Berko (1958) pioneered with children and which has subsequently used extensively in neuropsychological studies (see Table 1). In this task, a verb was presented in a given tense (e.g., present) and participants were instructed to produce the same verb in another tense (e.g., past). For example, for the Spanish sentence "*Hoy yo bebo, ayer yo ...*" [Today I drink, yesterday I ...], the expected response was the Spanish past-tense verb "*bebía*" [drank]. The sentences were spoken by the experimenter, and JM and MP gave their responses orally. The verbs were presented either in the present tense or past tense (see examples in Table 1) and the target responses involved producing verbs in the "other tense" (present or past). Verbs from each of the three conjugations were represented among the regular and irregular verbs tested in Spanish and Catalan. Different verbs were used in the two languages in order to create lists containing regular and irregular verbs as well as verbs from different conjugations.

Table 2 reports the results obtained with JM and MP in Spanish and Catalan. Both individuals were significantly less accurate with irregular vs regular verbs in each of their languages. The same result pattern was replicated with smaller sets of verbs matched for frequency, concreteness, and imageability (also see Table 2). The similarity across languages with regard to accuracy differences between regular and

TABLE 1

Materials used in the elicitation task to elicit regular and irregular inflections in Spanish and Catalan

	Eliciting sentence	Expected response
I. Spanish		
a. Past tense response		
Regular verb	Hoy yo bebo. Ayer yo _____ [Today I drink, yesterday I____ (drank)]	(bebia)
Irregular verb	Hoy yo voy. Ayer yo _____ [Today I go, yesterday I____ (went)]	(iba)
b. Present tense response		
Regular verb	Ayer yo miraba. Hoy yo ____ [Yesterday I looked, today I____ (look)]	(miro)
Irregular verb	Ayer yo daba. Hoy yo _____ [Yesterday I gave, today I____ (give)]	(doy)

TABLE 2
Results for the production of regular and irregular verb inflections in Spanish and Catalan: JM and MP

| | % (N) correct responses | | | |
| | Spanish | | Catalan | |
Participant	Regular	Irregular	Regular	Irregular
JM (L1 Spanish)				
	82% (28/34)	43% (13/30)*** [1]	91% (31/34)	72% (28/39)**
Matched subset[1]	82% (28/34)	55% (11/20)**	93% (28/30)	73% (22/30)**
MP (L1 Catalan)				
	89% (25/28)	52% (13/25)***	80% (28/35)	39% (7/18)***
Matched subset[2]	89% (16/18)	61% (11/18)*	86% (12/14)	45% (5/11)

[1] p values for the χ^2 statistics: * = $p < .01$, ** = $p < .05$, *** = $p < .01$.   [2] This list contained a subset of the regular and irregular verbs, which were matched for frequency, concreteness, and imageability.

irregular verb forms suggests a common underlying deficit in lexical/morphological retrieval for the two languages.

A German–English bilingual individual exhibiting a similar pattern of greater difficulties with irregular vs regular verbs in his two languages was reported by Cholin et al. (2007). A native speaker of German, WRG acquired English at the age of 8, when he began his schooling in English. Eventually WRG moved to the US, where he completed law school and pursed a career as a certified public accountant. WRG continued to use German regularly with relatives and in reading. As described above for Spanish and Catalan, for German and English irregular verbs are not associated with predictable semantic or phonological features (Clahsen, 1999; Marcus, Brinkmann, Clahsen, Wiese, & Pinker, 1995). However, German is unlike English in that all verb forms have an inflectional affix, while English allows for uninflected (citation) forms (e.g., in the present tense, as in "I drive"). With regard to German, we limit our more detailed description to the past participle, the tense tested in the German version of the sentence completion task administered to WRG. The past participle of a German verb is formed adding a suffix to the verb stem. In addition, for the group of what are typically referred to as the regular verbs, the stems do not undergo any change in the past participle (or other tenses) and take the "regular" past participle suffix -t. What are generally referred to as irregular verbs deviate from this pattern in different ways (see Table 3). Some irregular verbs are not subject to stem change in the past participle, differing only from the regular verbs in that they take the "irregular" inflection -en in the past participle. Other irregular verbs undergo stem change in the past participle and take the irregular inflection -en. Another, small group of verbs change the stem but take the regular inflection -t. With regard to the stem changes themselves, these always involve the vowels of the verb stems and in a few cases also their consonants. Depending on their prosodic pattern, regular and irregular verbs may take the suffix -ge (however this feature is not crucial for the purposes of contrasting regular and irregular verb inflections).

Three different types of German past participles were tested in a German version of the sentence completion task we described above: regulars (no stem change, suffix -t), no-stem-change irregulars (suffix -en), and stem-change irregulars (suffix -en

TABLE 3
Types of German verbs and their stems that were used in testing WRG

		Infinitive	Past participle	
Verb type		Stem	Stem	Suffix
Regular	No stem change	fragen (to ask) frag	gefragt frag	-t
Irregular	No stem change[1]	raten (guess) rat	geraten rat	-en
	Stem change	fliegen (to fly) flieg	geflogen flog	-en
		brennen (to burn) brenn	gebrannt brann	-t

[1]We indicate here whether the past participle contains an infinitive stem (no stem change) or takes a different stem (stem change). Irregular, no stem change verbs take a different stem in other inflections (e.g., past tense).

or -t). The three sets of regular and irregular verbs used in this task were matched for the frequencies of their lemmas as well as for the frequencies of their past participles (surface frequencies) (frequency norms were from Baayen, Piepenbrock, & Van Rijin, 1993). WRG's preserved ability to repeat spoken words ensured that the verb stimuli were correctly perceived. In each trial, a verb was introduced in its present tense—either the first person singular or the second person singular—and WRG was instructed to orally produce the past participle form of the verb (see examples in Table 4). It should be noted that with this type of testing procedure, the correct stem is provided in the stimulus for verbs that do not undergo stem change (regular and

TABLE 4
Materials used in the elicitation task to elicit regular and irregular inflections in German and English

	Eliciting sentence	Expected Response
I. German		
Present, first person singular, eliciting verb; past participle response		
regular no stem change	Heute sage ich. Gestern habe ich _____ [Today I say. In the past I have]	(gesagt) [said]
irregular no stem change	Heute rate ich. Gestern habe ich _____ [Today I guess. In the past I have]	(geraten) [guessed]
irregular stem change	Heute breche ich. Gestern habe ich _____ [Today I break. In the past I have]	(gebrochen) [broken]
II. English		
Present, first person singular, eliciting verb; past tense response		
Regular verb	Today I walk. Yesterday I _____	(walked)
Irregular verb	Today I give. Yesterday I _____	(gave)
Present, first person singular, eliciting verb; past participle response		
Regular verb	Today I walk. In the past I have _____	(walked)
Irregular verb	Today I give. In the past I have _____	(given)

TABLE 5
Results for WRG's production of regular and irregular verb inflections in German and English

	% (N) Correct responses			
	Whole word		Stems	
A. *German verbs*				
No-stem change, suffix –*t*	63%	(142/224)	82%	(185/224)
No stem change, suffix –*en*	63%	(106/168)	84%	(142/168)
Stem change, suffix -*t* or –*en*	29%	(69/237)	34%	(81/237)
B. *English verbs*				
Regular	68%	(254/373)	93%	(346/373)
Irregular	26%	(72/279)	33%	(91/279)

the no-stem-change irregulars). This is also true in English with regard to the regular verbs.

The results of testing are summarised in Table 5[4] and indicate that WRG was far more accurate with verbs that did not require a stem change (63%; 248/392), relative to verbs that took a different stem in the past participle (29%; 69/237; $\chi^2 = 68.91$, $p < .001$). Whether no-stem change past participles took the suffix -*t* or -*en* did not affect WRG's responses, as evidenced by their identical accuracy rates (63%). The most significant factor determining accuracy was whether the responses required the lexical retrieval of the stem, with only 29% accuracy with these verbs. The same pattern was observed whether one considered whole word or stem accuracy only (see Table 5). Interestingly, WRG encountered similar difficulties with English verb inflections. In an English version of the task, the stimuli consisted of verbs in their present tense and WRG was asked to produce either their past tense or their past participle (see examples in Table 4). Regular and irregular verbs were matched for lemma and surface frequencies (Baayen et al., 1993). The results indicate that in English regular verbs were produced significantly more accurately (68%; 254/373) than irregular verbs (26%, 72/279; $\chi^2 = 169.71$, $p < .001$). As in German, this pattern was observed whether one considered whole word accuracy or just stem accuracy (see Table 5).

Detailed analyses of WRG's errors revealed further similarities between the two languages and shed more light on his responses. Some of the errors made by WRG with stem-change verbs consisted of adding the regular suffix to the infinitive

---

[4] As observed in other cases of language impairments (Blumstein, 1978; Romani & Calabrese, 1998), WRG had problems in articulating consonant clusters, particularly those with complex sonority profiles (e.g., pairs of obstruent consonants). These problems affected WRG responses to German and English inflections that required the addition of the coronals /t/ and /d/ and caused a worsening in sonority at the end of the word (Clements, 1990; Ladefoged, 1975). For example, in *slipped*, the addition of the suffix -*ed* generates a coda with two obstruents and a worsening of the sonority profile. These phonological difficulties were coped by WRG with the insertion of epentheses that reduced the phonological complexity. For example, for /slipt/ (*slipped*) WRG said /slipit/—here, the vowel insertion avoids the occurrence of adjacent obstruent consonants. These types of phonological repairs were observed both in English and German with WRG. Responses that contained these types of repairs were scored as correct, a choice motivated on two grounds: (a) it is quite clear that such repairs occurred when WRG attempted to inflect the words, and (b) we were more interested in determining whether the correct inflection was selected rather than the consequences of these phonological difficulties (see Goldberg, Cholin, Bertz, Rapp, & Miozzo, 2007, for a discussion of these responses).

stem—an example, in English "caught" was produced as "catched". These so-called regularisation errors accounted for 35% of WRG's responses to stem-change verbs both in English and German. This is a type of error we expect to observe if information about a verb's irregular status or form is not available and the default pattern (e.g., in English, infinitive stem +*ed*) is used to derive the verb inflection. However, in English WRG sometimes produced errors like /spad/ for *sped* or /mɛit/ for *met*. What is interesting about these responses is that, as would be expected for an irregular verb, there was no suffix and, furthermore there were vowel changes in the stem. Similar responses to irregular verbs were also observed in German. These errors suggest that although he was unable to retrieve the correct form for the irregular verbs, WRG could sometime access sufficient information that allowed him to recognise that a verb was irregular and, therefore, that it required a stem change and no suffix. Rarely, in either German (5%) or English (2%) did WRG select a suffix that did not occur in the past tense or past participle (e.g., "hopes" for *hoped*). This suggests that, unlike in other cases of language impairments (e.g., Badecker & Caramazza, 1991), WRG's errors were not primarily due to problems in selecting suffixes satisfying proper morphological features (e.g., tense or person) but rather that his errors resulted from failures to access the form of the suffix (e.g., in German: -*t* vs -*en*).

In sum, in all three cases we see a striking similarity across languages in the patterns of performance with irregular vs regular verbs in terms of accuracy and errors. The three cases can be understood as involving disruption either to processes required for the retrieval of word stems or to the representations/processes involved in specifying the morphological characteristics of words. As in the previous cases, the cross-language similarities suggest a deficit to lexical retrieval processes instantiated in neural substrates that are shared across languages. We discuss the implications of these findings in the final section of this paper.

FINAL REMARKS

The neuropsychological data we have reviewed here reveal that lexical impairments affecting word-form retrieval can occur with considerable selectivity and cross-linguistic similarity in proficient bilingual speakers. This pattern of findings is consistent with the hypothesis that there are shared, cross-language neural substrates that support: (a) the representation and processing of word forms from specific grammatical categories and (b) the retrieval of word-forms and/or morphological information. While it is logically possible that this pattern of findings could occur in a system in which each language is supported by distinct, language-specific neural substrates, this would require that these substrates be damaged very similarly. This should be an unlikely event, especially with the large lesions in the cases we have highlighted here. Admittedly, however, the number of detailed case studies of this type is still quite small and future research will be critical for resolving these issues. Also to be determined is the degree to which shared substrates are limited to languages that share morpho-phonological similarities as do the language pairs (Spanish/Catalan and English/German) that were involved in these cases.

Findings such as these, indicating common neural substrates for quite specific aspects of lexical processing, need to be integrated with the findings from psycholinguistic research indicating that bilingual lexicons operate with considerable independence (Costa et al., 1999; Roelofs, 2003). This work refers specifically to the functioning of the cognitive systems, and not to their neural instantiation. Nonetheless, the data that we have reviewed here may help us to constrain hypotheses regarding the manner in which the lexical systems are instantiated. For example, one possibility is that functionally distinct lexical systems could be instantiated in distinct neural substrates, while another is that they are instantiated in common substrates—at least at a macroscopic level—with mechanisms that allow for relatively segregated and independent recruitment of lexical information. The findings reviewed here would seem to favour the latter hypothesis. However, this raises questions regarding the manner in which information about the two languages can be distinguished within shared substrates, so that the content of the target language is correctly selected at any given point in time. Here too, multiple hypotheses have been entertained. Some have suggested that the elements of each language are explicitly tagged regarding their language membership (e.g., Roelofs, 2003), while another holds that attentional mechanisms may also direct and supervise the language choice (Fabbro, Peru, & Skrap, 1997; Green, 1998, 2005).

It is important to note that all of the cases we have reviewed have involved highly proficient bilingual people who have used both languages extensively since acquiring them. There are a number of results indicating that proficiency and age of acquisition may be highly relevant to the organisation of the bilingual brain. Therefore the conclusions reached here can only be extended to the highly proficient bilingual people who acquired their L2 in childhood. However, despite their great proficiency in both languages, it is also interesting that all of the bilingual individuals reviewed here acquired one language before the other; although, in all cases, L2 was learned during childhood, and each individual achieved an excellent control of L2 through a consistent and extensive use. These facts imply that primary features of the lexical organisation in L1, such as grammatical class distinctions and word inflections, can transfer to L2 even when the languages are not acquired simultaneously. Interestingly, Kambanaros and van Steenbrugge (2006) reported that verbs were more affected than nouns in both of the languages spoken by a group of *late* Greek–English bilingual speakers affected by anomia. As in the cases we have described here, these grammatical class deficits involved the retrieval of nouns/verbs rather than the meaning of actions/objects. Kambanaros and van Steenbrugge's results suggest that grammatical class distinctions can emerge even in bilingual people who acquired a second language as adults.

Despite the striking similarities across languages, it is worth pointing out that at least one of the individuals described in our review (JPG) exhibited significantly more severe disruption to verbs than nouns in his L2 (Catalan) than in his L1 (Spanish). The similarities between the nouns and verbs of Catalan and Spanish make it unlikely that JPG was less accurate in Catalan because of the greater complexity of the verb system in this language. It is possible that JPG's performance reflects some difference in the age of acquisition of the two languages, although clear L1/L2 differences were not observed in the other four cases despite the fact that the languages were acquired asynchronously. JPG's data further imply that despite their shared substrates, L1 and L2 are encoded in some manner that allows for their differential susceptibility to disruption.

Results such as these quite naturally raise the question of why different language-processing systems should share neural substrates. Hypotheses regarding this issue include Hernández et al.'s (2007) "language domain hypothesis" as well as Green's (2003) proposal of "convergence". According to these hypotheses, neural networks specialise for certain language functions (e.g., grammatical vs lexical processing) either because they are innately predetermined to take these functions (Hernandez et al., 2007) or because they respond to certain properties of language in an increasingly selective manner (Green, 2003). Once this form of specialisation is achieved for L1, it would also operate for L2. At present these types of accounts are only speculative, but will certainly serve to guide future research.

Finally, we would like to comment on the role played by associations in deficit patterns in developing theories of bilingual language processing. Just as has been pointed out in the development of theories of monolingual language processing (e.g., Hillis, Rapp, Romani, & Caramazza 1990; Woollams, Lambon Ralph, Plaut, & Patterson, 2007) while dissociations in performance across tasks and cognitive functions can be enormously informative, there may also much to be learned from patterns of associations of deficits, especially when they are highly specific and detailed. The approach adopted in these studies was to determine whether a selective deficit observed in one language (e.g., verbs vs nouns) occurred in the other language. We hoped to have shown that seeking similarities in patterns of breakdown across languages can be a productive approach to furthering our understanding of the bilingual brain.

REFERENCES

Abutalebi, J., Cappa, S. F., & Perani, D. (2001). The bilingual brain as revealed by functional imaging. *Bilingualism: Language and Cognition, 4*, 179–190.

Abutalebi, J., & Green, D. (2007). Bilingual language production: The neurocognition of language representation and control. *Journal of Neurolinguistics, 20*, 242–275.

Abutalebi, J., Miozzo, A., & Cappa, S. F. (2000). Do subcortical structures control language selection in bilinguals? Evidence from pathological language mixing. *Neurocase, 6*, 101–106.

Aglioti, S., Beltramello, A., Girardi, F., & Fabbro, F. (1996). Neurolinguistic and follow-up study of an unusual pattern of recovery from bilingual subcortical aphasia. *Brain, 119*, 1151–1564.

Albert, M. L., & Obler, L. K. (1978). *The bilingual brain: Neuropsychological and neurolinguistic aspects of bilingualism.* New York: Academic Press.

Almagro, Y., Sanchez-Casa, R., & Garcia-Albea, J. E. (2003). Estudio de un caso de anomia: Efectos de la categoria grammatical en la production de un afasico bilinguies [A case study of anomia: Grammatical category in the production of a bilingual aphasic.] *Cognitiva, 15*, 33–49.

Baayen, R., Piepenbrock, R., & Van Rijin, H. (1993). *The CELEX lexical database.* Philadelphia, PA: Linguistic Data Consortium, University of Pennsylvania.

Badecker, W., & Caramazza, A. (1991). Morphological composition in the lexical output system. *Cognitive Neuropsychology, 8*, 335–367.

Badecker, W., Miozzo, M., & Zanuttini, R. (1997). The two-stage model of lexical retrieval: Evidence of a case of anomia with selective preservation of grammatical gender. *Cognition, 57*, 193–216.

Berko, J. (1958). The child's learning of English morphology. *Word, 14*, 150–177.

Berlingeri, M., Crepaldi, D., Roberti, R., Scialfa, G., Luzzatti, C., & Paulesu, E. (2008). Nouns and verbs in the brain: Grammatical class and task specific effects as revealed by fMRI. *Cognitive Neuropsychology, 25*, 528–554.

Bird, H., Howard, D., & Franklin, S. (2000). Why is a verb like an inanimate object? Grammatical category and semantic category deficits. *Brain and Language, 72*, 246–309.

Blumstein, S. E. (1978). Segment structure and the syllable in aphasia. In A. Bell & J. B. Hooper (Eds.), *Syllables and segments* (pp. 189–200). The Netherlands: North Holland.

Caramazza, A., & Hillis, A. E. (1991). Lexical organisation of nouns and verbs in the brain. *Nature, 349*, 788–790.

Chee, M. W. L., Hon, N., Lee, H. L., & Soon, C. S. (2001). Relative language proficiency modulates BOLD signal change when bilinguals perform semantic judgments. *Neuroimage, 13*, 1155–1163.

Chee, M. W., Soon, C. S., Lee, H. L., & Pallier, C. (2004). Left insula activation: A marker for language attainment in bilinguals. *Proceedings of the National Academy of Sciences, U.S.A.*, *101*, 15265–15270.

Cholin, J., Goldberg, A. M., Bertz, J. W., Rapp, B., & Miozzo, M. (2007). The nature of the processing distinction between regular and irregular verbs: Evidence from an English–German bilingual aphasic speaker. *Brain and Language*, *103*, 61–62.

Clahsen, H. (1999). Lexical entries and rules of language: A multidisciplinary study of German inflections. *Behavioural and Brain Sciences*, *22*, 991–1060.

Clements, G. N. (1990). The role of sonority cycle in core syllabification. In J. Kingston & M. E. Beckam (Eds.), *Papers in laboratory phonology I: Between the grammar and the physics of speech*. Cambridge, UK: Cambridge University Press.

Cortese, M. J., Balota, D. A., Sergent-Marshall, S. D., Buckner, R. L., & Gold, B. T. (2006). Consistency and regularity in past-tense verb generation in healthy ageing, Alzheimer's disease, and semantic dementia. *Cognitive Neuropsychology*, *23*, 856–876.

Costa, A., Caramazza, A., & Sebastián-Gallés, N. (2000). The cognate facilitation effect: Implications for models of lexical access. *Journal of Experimental Psychology: Learning, Memory, and Cognition*, *26*, 1283–1296.

Costa, A., Miozzo, M., & Caramazza, A. (1999). Lexical selection in bilinguals: Do words in bilingual's lexicon compete for selection? *Journal of Memory and Language*, *41*, 365–397.

Costa, A., Santesban, M., & Caño, A. (2005). On the facilitatory effects of cognate words in bilingual speech production. *Brain and Language*, *94*, 94–103.

De Bleser, R., Dupont, P., Postler, J., Bormans, G., Mortelmans, L., & Debrock, M. (2003). The organisation of the bilingual lexicon: A PET study. *Journal of Neurolinguistics*, *16*, 439–456.

de Diego Balaguer, R., Costa, A., Sebastián-Gallés, N., Juncadella, M., & Caramazza, A. (2004). Regular and irregular morphology and its relationship with agrammatism: Evidence from two Spanish–Catalan bilinguals. *Brain and Language*, *91*, 212–222.

Dehaene, S., Dupoux, E., Mehler, J., Cohen, L., Paulesu, E., & Perani, D. (1997). Anatomical variability in the cortical representation of first and second languages. *Neuroreport*, *8*, 3809–3815.

Fabbro, F., Peru, A., & Skrap, M. (1997). Language disorders in bilingual patients after thalamic lesions. *Journal of Neurolinguistics*, *10*, 347–367.

García-Caballero, A., García-Lado, I., González-Hermida, J., Area, R., Recimil, M. J., & Juncos Rabandán, O., et al. (2007). Paradoxical recovery in a bilingual patient with aphasia after right capsuloputaminal infarction. *Journal of Neurology, Neurosurgery, and Psychiatry*, *78*, 89–91.

Goldberg, A. M., Cholin, J., Bertz, J. W., Rapp, B., & Miozzo, M. (2007). Evidence for morpho-phonological processes in spoken production. *Brain and Language*, *103*, 162–163.

Gollan, T. H., & Acenas, L. R. (2004). GAT is a TOT? Cognate and translation effects on tip-of-the-tongue states in Spanish–English and Tagalog–English bilinguals. *Journal of Experimental Psychology: Learning, Memory, and Cognition*, *30*, 246–269.

Gollan, T. H., & Kroll, J. F. (2001). Bilingual lexical access. In B. Rapp (Ed.), *The handbook of cognitive neuropsychology* (pp. 321–345). Philadelphia, PA: Psychology Press.

Gomez-Tortosa, E., Martin, E., Gaviria, M., Charbel, F., & Ausma, J. (1995). Selective deficit in one language in a bilingual patient following surgery in the left perisylvian area. *Brain and Language*, *48*, 320–325.

Green, D. W. (1986). Control, activation and resource: A framework and a model for the control of speech in bilinguals. *Brain and Language*, *27*, 210–223.

Green, D. W. (1998). Mental control of the bilingual lexico-semantic system. *Bilingualism: Language and Cognition*, *1*, 67–81.

Green, D. W. (2003). The neural basis of the lexicon and the grammar in L2 acquisition. In R. van Hout, A. Hulk, F. Kuiken, & R. Towell (Eds.), *The interface between syntax and the lexicon in second language acquisition*. Amsterdam: John Benjamins.

Green, D. W. (2005). The neurocognition of recovery patterns in bilingual aphasics. In J. F. Kroll & A. M. B. de Groot (Eds.), *Handbook of bilingualism: Psycholinguistic approaches* (pp. 516–530). New York: Oxford University Press.

Green, D. W., & Abutalebi, J. (in press). Understanding the link between bilingual aphasia and language control. *Acta Psychologica*.

Green, D. W., Crinion, J., & Price, C. J. (2006). Convergence, divergence and control. *Language Learning*, *56*, 99–125.

Greenberg, J. (1976). *Language universals*. The Hague: Mouton.

Hermans, D., Bongaerts, T., De Bot, K., & Scheuder, R. (1998). Producing words in a foreign language: Can speakers prevent interference from their first language? *Bilingualism: Language and Cognition, 1*, 213–229.

Hernandez, A. E., Dapretto, M., Mazziotta, J., & Bookheimer, S. (2001). Language switching and language representation in Spanish–English bilinguals. *Neuroimage, 14*, 510–520.

Hernández, M., Caño, A., Costa, A., Sebastián-Gallés, N., Juncadella, M., & Gascón-Bayarri, J. (2008). Grammatical category-specific deficits in bilingual aphasia. *Brain and Language, 107*, 68–80.

Hernández, M., Costa, A., Sebastián-Gallés, N., Juncadella, M., & Reñe, R. (2007). The organisation of nouns and verbs in bilingual speakers: A case of bilingual grammatical category-specific deficit. *Journal of Neurolinguistics, 20*, 285–305.

Hillis, A. E. (2001). The organisation of the lexical system. In B. Rapp (Ed.), *The handbook of cognitive neuropsychology* (pp. 185–210). Philadelphia, PA: Psychology Press.

Hillis, A. E., Rapp, B., Romani, C., & Caramazza, A. (1990). Selective impairments of semantics in lexical processing. *Cognitive Neuropsychology, 7*, 191–243.

Hillis, A. E., Tuffiash, E., & Caramazza, A. (2002). Modality-specific deterioration in naming verbs in nonfluent primary progressive aphasia. *Journal of Cognitive Neuroscience, 14*, 1099–1108.

Indefrey, P. (2006). A meta-analysis of hemodynamic studies on first and second language processing: Which suggested differences can we trust and what do they mean? *Language Learning, 56*, 279–304.

Joanisse, M. F., & Seidenberg, M. S. (1999). Impairments in verb morphology after brain injury: A connectionist model. *Proceedings of the National Academy of Sciences, 96*, 7592–7597.

Kambanaros, M., & van Steenbrugge, W. (2006). Noun and verb processing in Greek–English bilingual individuals with anomic aphasia and the effect of instrumentality and verb–noun relation. *Brain and Language, 97*, 162–177.

Kay, J., & Ellis, A. (1987). A cognitive neuropsychological case study of anomia. *Brain, 110*, 613–629.

Klein, D., Watkins, K. E., Zatorre, R. J., & Milner, B. (2006). Word and nonword repetition in bilingual subjects: A PET study. *Human Brain Mapping, 27*, 153–161.

Kirsner, K., Smith, M. C., Lockhart, R. L. S., King, M. L., & Jain, M. (1984). The bilingual lexicon: Language-specific units in an integrated network. *Journal of Verbal Learning and Verbal Behavior, 23*, 519–539.

Kovelman, I., Baker, S. A., & Petitto, L-A. (2008). Bilingual ad monolingual brains compared: A functional magnetic resonance imaging investigation of syntactic processing and a possible "neural signature" of bilingualism. *Journal of Cognitive Neuroscience, 20*, 153–169.

Kroll, J. F., & Stewart, E. (1994). Category interference in translation and picture naming: Evidence for asymmetric connections between bilingual memory representations. *Journal of Memory and Language, 33*, 149–174.

Kroll, J. F., & Tokowicz, N. (2005). Models of bilingual representation and processing. In *Handbook of bilingualism: Psycholinguistic approaches* (pp. 531–553). New York: Oxford University Press.

Ladefoged, P. (1975). *A course in phonetics*. New York: Harcourt, Brace, Jovanovich.

La Heij, W., De Bruyn, E., Elens, E., Hartsuiker, R., Helaha, D., & Van Schelven, L. (1990). Orthographic facilitation and categorical interference in a word-translation variant of the Stroop task. *Canadian Journal of Psychology, 44*, 76–83.

Lambon-Ralph, M. A., Sage, K., & Roberts, J. (2000). Classical anomia: A neuropsychological perspective on speech production. *Neuropsychologia, 38*, 186–202.

Lucas, T. H., McKhann, G. M., & Ojemann, G. A. (2004). Functional separation of languages in bilingual brain: A comparison of electrical stimulation language mapping in 25 bilingual patients and 117 monolingual control patients. *Journal of Neurosurgery, 101*, 449–457.

Malt, B. C., Sloman, S. A., Gennari, S., Shi, M., & Wang, Y. (1999). Knowing versus naming: similarity and the linguistic categorization of artifacts. *Journal of Memory and Language, 40*, 230–262.

Marcus, G. F. (2000). *The algebric mind: Reflections on connectionism and cognitive science*. Cambridge, MA: MIT Press.

Marcus, G. F., Brinkmann, U., Clahsen, H., Wiese, R., & Pinker, S. (1995). German inflection: The exception that proves the rule. *Cognitive Psychology, 29*, 189–256.

Marshall, J., Chiat, S., Robson, J., & Pring, T. (1996a). Calling a salad a federation: An investigation of semantic jargon. Part 2 – Verbs. *Journal of Neurolinguistics, 9*, 251–260.

Marshall, J., Pring, T., Chiat, S., & Robson, J. (1996b). Calling a salad a federation: An investigation of semantic jargon. Part 1 – Nouns. *Journal of Neurolinguistics, 9,* 237–250.

Miceli, G., Turriziani, P., Caltagirone, C., Capasso, R., Tomaiuolo, F., & Caramazza, A. (2002). The neural correlates of grammatical gender: An fMRI investigation. *Journal of Cognitive Neuroscience, 14,* 618–628.

Miozzo, M. (2003). On the processing of regular and irregular forms of verbs and nouns: Evidence from neuropsychology. *Cognition, 87,* 101–127.

Miozzo, M., & Caramazza, A. (1997). On knowing the auxiliary of a verb that cannot be named. *Journal of Cognitive Neuroscience, 9,* 160–166.

Miozzo, M., & Gordon, P. (2005). Facts, events, and inflection: When language and memory dissociate. *Journal of Cognitive Neuroscience, 17,* 1074–1086.

Ojemann, G. A. (1995). Awake operations with mapping in epilepsy. In H. H. Schmidek & W. H. Sweet (Eds.), *Operative neurosurgical techniques: Indications, methods and results, 3rd ed* (pp. 1317–1322). Philadelphia: W. B. Saunders.

Paradis, M. (1977). The cognitive neuropsychology of bilingualism. In H. Whitaker & H. A. Whitaker (Eds.), *Studies in neurolinguistics* (pp. 65–121). New York: Academic Press.

Paradis, M. (1998). Language and communication in multilinguals. In B. Stemmer & H. Whitaker (Eds.), *Handbook of neurolinguistics* (pp. 417–430). San Diego, CA: Academic Press.

Paradis, M. (2001). Bilingual and polyglot aphasia. In R. S. Berndt (Ed.), *Handbook of neuropsychology* (pp. 69–91). Amsterdam: Elsevier Science.

Parris, B., & Weekes, B. (2001). Action naming in dementia. *Neurocase, 7,* 459–471.

Patterson, K., Lambon Ralph, M. A., Hodges, J. R., & McClelland, J. L. (2001). Deficits in irregular past-tense verb morphology associated with degraded semantic knowledge. *Neuropsychologia, 39,* 709–724.

Penke, M., Janssen, U., & Krause, M. (1999). The representation of inflectional morphology: Evidence from Broca's aphasia. *Brain and Language, 68,* 225–232.

Perani, D., Abutalebi, J., Paulesu, E., Scifo, P., Cappa, S. F., & Fazio, F. (2003). The role of age of acquisition and language use in early, high proficient bilinguals: A fMRI study during verbal fluency. *Human Brain Mapping, 19,* 170–182.

Pinker, S. (1991). Rules of language. *Science, 253,* 530–533.

Pitres, A. (1895). Etude sur l'aphasie chez les polyglottes. *Revue de médecine, 15,* 873–899. [Translated in M. Paradis (Ed.), (1983). *Readings on aphasia in bilinguals and polyglots* (pp. 26–48). Montreal: Marcel Didier.].

Potter, M. C., Von Eckardt, B., & Feldman, L. B. (1984). Lexical and conceptual representations in beginning and more proficient bilinguals. *Journal of Verbal Learning and Verbal Behavior, 23,* 23–38.

Rapp, B., & Caramazza, A. (1998). A case of selective difficulty in writing verbs. *Neurocase, 4,* 127–140.

Rapp, B., & Goldrick, M. (2006). Speaking words: The contribution of cognitive neuropsychological research. *Cognitive Neuropsychology, 23,* 39–73.

Roberts, P. M., & Deslauriers, L. (1999). Picture naming of cognate and non-cognate nouns in bilingual aphasia. *Journal of Communication Disorders, 32,* 1–23.

Robinson, K. M., Grossman, M., White-Devine, T., & D'Esposito, M. (1996). Category-specific difficulty naming with verbs in Alzheimer's disease. *Neurology, 47,* 178–182.

Roelofs, A. (2003). Goal-oriented selection of verbal action: Modeling attentional control in the Stroop Task. *Psychological Review, 110,* 88–125.

Romani, C., & Calabrese, A. (1998). Syllabic constraints in the phonological errors of an aphasic patient. *Brain and Language, 64,* 83–121.

Rumelhart, D. E., & McClelland, J. L. (1986). On learning the past tenses of English verbs. In J. L. McClelland, D. E. Rumelhart, & PDP Research Group (Eds.), *Parallel distributed processing: Explorations in the microstructure of cognition. Vol 1. Foundations.* Cambridge, MA: MIT Press.

Shapiro, K., Shelton, J., & Caramazza, A. (2000). Grammatical class in lexical production and morphological processing: Evidence from a case of fluent aphasia. *Cognitive Neuropsychology, 17,* 665–670.

Stowe, L., & Sabouring, L. (2005). Imaging the processing of a second language: Effects of maturation and proficiency on neural processes involved. *International Review of Applied Linguistics in Language Teaching, 43,* 329–354.

Tyler, L. K., Randall, B., & Marslen-Wilson, W. D. (2002). Phonology and morphology of the English past tense. *Neuropsychologia, 40,* 1154–1166.

Ullman, M. T. (2001). A neurocognitive perspective on language: The declarative/procedural model. *Nature Reviews Neuroscience, 2,* 717–726.

Ullman, M. T., Corkin, S., Coppola, M., Hickok, G., Growdon, J. H., & Koroshetz, W. J. et al. (1997). A neural dissociation within language: Evidence that the mental dictionary is part of declarative memory, and that grammatical rules are processed by the procedural system. *Journal of Cognitive Neuroscience*, *9*, 266–276.

Ullman, M. T., & Gopnik, M. (1999). Inflectional morphology in a family with inherited specific language impairment. *Applied Psycholinguistics*, *20*, 51–117.

Warterburger, I., Heekeren, H. R., Abutalebi Cappa, S. F., Villringer, A., & Perani, D. (2003). Early setting of grammatical processing in the bilingual brain. *Neuron*, *37*, 159–170.

Woollams, A. M., Lambon Ralph, M. A., Plaut, D. C., & Patterson, K. (2007). SD-squared: On the association between semantic dementia and surface dyslexia. *Psychological Review*, *114*, 316–339.

Zingeser, L. B., & Berndt, R. S. (1988). Grammatical class and context effects in a case of pure anomia: Implications for models of language production. *Cognitive Neuropsychology*, *5*, 473–516.

APPENDIX: BACKGROUND INFORMATION ON INDIVIDUALS DISCUSSED IN THE PAPER

LPM

LPM was a Catalan–Spanish bilingual woman who worked mostly as a seamstress until her retirement. She was born in Barcelona, where Catalan and Spanish are both official languages. LPM acquired Catalan as her L1, using it at home (first with her parents and siblings, later with her husband and children), at work, and in several other daily activities. LPM started to speak Spanish, her L2, early in her life with one of the relatives who lived in her house as well as with her parents and siblings. LPM received her education in Spanish and used this language in everyday contexts. LPM was 74 years old when she participated in the research study.

LPM was diagnosed with AD in September 2005. At this time, LPM's disease was mild in severity, allowing her to continue living on her own and taking care of basic chores. Needing help for more complex activities, she was regularly supervised by one of her daughters. The experience of frequent tip-of-the-tongue states was the major complaint reported by LPM and her family, as these word-finding failures severely limited her communication in everyday situations such as shopping. The neuropsychological examination revealed that LPM's spontaneous speech was fluent with no grammatical errors. However, moderate anomia affected LPM's speaking in both languages. Other language functions such as comprehension, repetition, reading, and writing to dictation were relatively preserved. Testing of praxis and gnosis were within normal range, and episodic memory was relatively spared. SPECT revealed severe hypoperfusion in left temporal regions as well as global cortical atrophy.

JPG

JPG was a Spanish–Catalan bilingual architect, who was born in Barcelona in 1948. His L1 was Spanish, the language that he used with his parents and siblings, and in which he received his education. JPG acquired Catalan (L2) before the age of 4 by using it with other relatives, schoolmates, and friends. Some of JPG's university courses were taught in Catalan. JPG regularly used Catalan with his wife and daughter, and at work. As reported by his wife, JPG had a native-level of proficiency in Catalan since childhood.

JPG was diagnosed with PPA in 2002 at the age of 54. His main symptoms consisted of disinhibited behaviour and frequent tip-of-the-tongue states. With the onset of the illness JPG stopped using Catalan, even with his wife and daughter with whom he had routinely conversed in this language. The neuropsychological examination revealed oral and written difficulties both in L1 and L2, anomias, and phonological errors. No other neuropsychological deficits were detected during this initial stage of the disease. The MRI scans obtained as JPG's illness progressed showed signs of cerebral atrophy that became increasingly evident in the prefrontal, anterior temporal, and insular areas. In 2003, as the severity of JPG's disease progressed to moderate stages, his spontaneous speech became less fluent and more agrammatic, ultimately reducing to automatisms such as "yes", "no", and "eh". JPG's executive functions, including mental flexibility and planning, also gradually worsened. Other language abilities, including comprehension, repetition, writing to dictation, and reading, remained relatively spared. JPG showed increasingly severe difficulties in oral and writing naming, and at every stage of the disease, L2 (Catalan) appeared to be more affected than L1 (Spanish).

JM

JM was a Spanish–Catalan bilingual man with college education, who suffered a haemorrhagic stroke at the age of 50 years (9 years before participating in the research study). A SPECT conducted in 2002 revealed cerebral hypoperfusion, which was severe in the frontal lobe, moderate in the parietal lobe, and mild in the temporal lobe. An MRI scan carried out at the same time showed abnormalities in the left frontotemporal subcortical area and periventricular right hemisphere.

Spanish was JM's L1 and the language in which he received his education both in school and college. JM had used Catalan (L2) on daily basis since childhood. JM's conversations with his wife and son occurred in Catalan and JM reported preferring to speak this language. L1 and L2 appeared to be affected to a similar extent by JM's stroke. JM's spontaneous speech was non-fluent, anomic, and with frequent subject-agreement errors. Omissions and substitutions of verbs and function words (especially propositions) were also noticeable. Some of JM's errors with verbs consisted of semantically related substitutions or intrusions from his other language. JM also had articulatory difficulties that made him perform poorly in word repetition and reading.

JM's picture naming was similarly impaired in both languages and most of JM's errors were accounted for by circumlocutions, non-responses, or morphological errors. Although JM's word comprehension seemed to be relatively spared, his sentence comprehension was impaired, especially with passive sentences and when tested with materials in which thematic roles were reversed. Similar difficulties with passive forms and thematic role assignment were observed in sentence production.

MP

MP was a Catalan–Spanish bilingual woman with college education, who had a left temporal hematoma as a consequence of an aneurysm at the trifurcation of the left middle cerebral artery. SPECT conducted at time of the research study, when MP was 42 years old and 7 years after the brain lesion, showed marked hypoactivity in the entire left hemisphere.

MP was first exposed to Catalan (L1), although she acquired Spanish (L2) at an early age and received education in this language. MP's languages appeared to be affected to a similar extent by the brain damage. Her spontaneous language was non-fluent, anomic, with omissions of verbs, and omissions and substitutions of prepositions and other function words. Sentences were often left incomplete and contained agreement violations involving verbs, particularly their tense and person. Occasionally, MP also produced errors in which nouns and verbs were substituted by phonologically or semantically related words.

MP performed well in oral repetition tasks, and was better in reading words than non-words in both languages, mostly making phonological errors in non-word reading. Word comprehension, as tested with word–picture matching tasks, was intact. Sentence comprehension was mildly impaired in the two languages with active sentences and passive sentences. MP's sentence comprehension worsened for materials in which thematic roles were reversed.

WRG

WRG was born in Germany and German was his native language. At the age of 8, WRG moved to China where he lived until the age of 18, attending an international, English-speaking school. WRG then moved to the US where he earned a college degree and a degree in law and, until his retirement, worked as a certified public accountant. English became his dominant language, speaking it daily at home and at work. He maintained his German by speaking with his family and reading in German regularly. In July 2004 he suffered a stroke that produced damage in the area of the distribution of the left middle and posterior cerebral arteries. The research study started 2 years after his stroke, when he was 76, and continued for about a year. During this time his condition remained stable. WRG's language impairment had similar characteristics in English and German. The Aachen Aphasie Test, AAT (Huber, Poeck, Weniger, & Willmes, 1983) was used to assess WRG's language impairment in German.

WRG's spontaneous speech was reduced to short effortful utterances. WRG's lexical access was impaired in speaking, as evidenced by his difficulties in naming pictures of common objects. Most of WRG's naming errors were neologisms that had little resemblance to the target word, in addition to perseverations, phonologically related responses, and occasional semantically related responses. WRG's spoken word comprehension was relatively good in English—standard score of 98 (45th percentile) in PPVT, Form L—but slightly worse in German (5/10 correct responses). Grammatical processing was tested in English and WRG was able to correctly judge the grammaticality of 8/10 sentences that were presented auditorily and to complete 8/10 (80%) sentences producing the correct prepositions or phrases. Oral reading was impaired in German (7/10 correct responses) and English (42/40 correct responses; with no difference in accuracy between words with regular and irregular spelling). Although letter writing and word copying were preserved, writing words to dictation was impaired—correct responses: 4/20 (20%) in English, 0/10 in German. Some of WRG's spelling errors were phonologically plausible realisations of the word (*dance* → DANSE); others included multiple incorrect letters (e.g., *toss* → TOWL).

APHASIOLOGY, 2010, 24 (2), 288–308

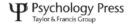

Executive function and conversational strategies in bilingual aphasia

Claire Penn, Tali Frankel, Jennifer Watermeyer, and Nicole Russell

University of the Witwatersrand, Johannesburg, South Africa

Background: Deficits of executive function (EF) have been proposed as all or part of the underlying mechanisms of language impairment in at least some types of aphasia. Executive functions also play a role in the recovery process. There is evidence that bilingual persons have some executive functioning advantages compared to monolingual persons. In this paper we combine two lines of recent investigation in order to explore the relationship between executive function and conversational strategies in bilingual aphasia.
Aims: The aim of this preliminary research was to compare the executive functioning profiles of bilingual individuals to those of monolingual participants with aphasia. A further aim was to examine evidence in the conversational samples of the participants in relation to the application of a range of executive skills and to link cognitive and conversational profiles using Barkley's (1997) model of executive functions.
Methods & Procedures: The performance of two bilingual individuals with aphasia on a test battery of executive function tests was compared with that of eight monolingual persons (seven with aphasia and one with right hemisphere damage). The test battery included measures of behavioural inhibition, working memory, problem solving, and reconstitution. The presence or absence of executive features in the conversational samples of the participants was judged by four raters using conversational analysis methods.
Outcomes & Results: Significant differences were found between the scores of the bilingual participants and those of the monolingual participants on measures of behavioural inhibition, working memory, planning and problem solving, and reconstitution. The bilingual participants' scores were mostly within normal limits and suggested well-retained executive functions. Conversation analysis showed evidence of differential application of these executive functions to conversational management. Regardless of severity or type of aphasia, the bilingual participants showed evidence of good topic management, repair, and flexibility compared to the monolingual participants.
Conclusions: The results are interpreted in relation to current issues in bilingualism. Our preliminary findings shed light on differential approaches to assessment, therapy, and choice of language for bilingual aphasia.

Keywords: Executive function; Bilingual aphasia; Language treatment; Compensatory strategies; Conversation analysis.

Address correspondence to: Claire Penn, Department of Speech Pathology and Audiology, University of the Witwatersrand, Private Bag 3, Wits 2050, Johannesburg, South Africa. E-mail: claire.penn@ wits.ac.za

The authors would like to thank Peter Fridjhon for his assistance with statistical analysis. This project was funded by scholarships from Deutscher Akademischer Austausch Dienst, National Research Foundation, and University of the Witwatersrand.

http://www.psypress.com/aphasiology   DOI: 10.1080/02687030902958399

Bilingualism provides certain advantages to the user of language in context. It provides the opportunity to shift languages and to interact with a range of persons. It allows for flexibility of choice and thus serves as a window not just into linguistic processes but also onto cognitive and pragmatic aspects. Regardless of the type of bilingualism and language, the bilingual language user usually has a choice to bear within certain contexts and can exercise that choice. The context can thus serve to prime both the exercising of choice and the language act itself.

There has been considerable research on whether there are special cognitive characteristics in the bilingual language user. If, as suggested by Goral, Levy, Obler, and Cohen (2006) and Crinion et al. (2006), there is overlapping cortical language representation at least for highly proficient bilingual people and both languages are activated when a person uses one of them, then attention to the selected language must be controlled and the non-targeted language must be inhibited (Bialystok, Craik, Grady, Chau, & Ishii, 2005). Executive control tasks are therefore enhanced in bilingual people because of their constant involvement in language use (Bialystok, 2007). Some of the evidence from child language supports this view. Bialystok (1999) for example points out that bilingual children consistently perform better in tasks demanding high levels of cognitive control, and that these children are better able to resist distraction and control their attention than their monolingual peers. In relation to disordered language, this research has extended into the field of both child language disorders and aphasia. The suggestion has been made that there may be more flexibility in the bilingual brain for coping with context. If this is the case then we might expect to see such flexibility emerge even under conditions of acquired language impairment. The present paper explores this notion in relation to brain damage by comparing the executive and conversation profiles of bilingual versus monolingual persons with acquired language impairment.

Some symptoms of bilingual aphasia, such as code switching and other grammatical and discourse behaviours that have been interpreted as direct symptoms of an underlying linguistic deficit, may actually arise from the interactional context in which they are produced (Beeke, Wilkinson, & Maxim, 2003a, 2003b; Fabbro, Skrap, & Agliotti, 2000; Ogilvy, von Bentheim, Venter, Ulatowska, & Penn, 2000; Penn, 2007) and this may reflect adaptation, compensation, shift, and flexibility, which are components of executive functioning (EF). These behaviours thus appear to represent an attempt to manage sequential demands of talk within the confines of aphasia, i.e., to adapt to the structural demands of conversation. Such a formulation of compensatory shift relies heavily on environmental priming, which in the case of bilingual patients will include the language environment of the speech act. As research has demonstrated, compensatory shift also appears to depend on the underlying neurological substrates and specifically on executive function.

One question that arises from this research is whether this capacity to shift can be measured formally and whether this has any correlates in neuropsychological testing. The success of compensation may link to the application of underlying executive processes in context. This paper will focus on some of the features of conversation that suggest the active use of compensatory strategies and will explore whether bilingualism offers an advantage in this regard.

Evidence of executive dysfunction in individuals with aphasia has been provided by several sources. A body of recent research suggests, for example, that deficits in cognitive effort or intention may be implicated as potential contributors to the communication problems in aphasia (Crosson et al., 2005; Korda & Douglas, 1997; McNeil et al., 2004; Owen, Downes, Sahakian, Polkey, & Robbins, 1990; Purdy, 2002; Rende, 2000). For example, Korda and Douglas (1997) demonstrated deficits in attentional capacity in 21 stroke patients with slower processing speed and greater increases in response time in a series of reaction time tasks. Similarly Lindfield, Polzik, and Roberts (2000) demonstrated deficits in both long-term and short-term memory, independent of language deficits in individuals with aphasia. Villiard (1990) attributed agrammatism to underlying attention and working memory deficits. Murray and colleagues (Murray, 2000; Murray, Holland, & Beeson, 1998) found that word-finding deficits were related to deficits in divided and focused attention. The reduced ability of a group of individuals with anterior left hemisphere lesions and co-occurring memory difficulties to recall a list of semantically related words was attributed to difficulty retrieving relevant categories from long-term episodic memory. Murray et al.'s work (1998) also suggests that attentional demands may have a negative impact on spoken language in people with mild aphasia.

Executive function also plays a role in recovery from aphasia (Bailey, Powell, & Clark, 1981; Coelho, 2005; Helm-Estabrooks, Tabor Connor, & Albert, 2000; Ramsberger, 2005; Sturm, Willmes, Orgass, & Hartje, 1997). Differential profiles of recovery have been identified and evidence suggests a link between better communication skills and better retained or recovered EF (Miyake, Emerson, & Friedman, 2000; Purdy, 1992). Similarly, improvements in aspects of language performance are associated with attention and executive training programmes (Coelho, 2005; Helm-Estabrooks et al., 2000; Ramsberger, 2005).

Advanced neuroimaging has demonstrated that executive functions are located in different parts of the brain from language areas and that cognitive control emerges from the interaction of separable neural systems. Executive functions are primarily associated with the prefrontal cortex and its reciprocal connections (Abutalebi & Green, 2007; Crinion et al., 2006). The differential recovery of aphasia in response to therapy and the failure to apply suitable compensatory strategies to real-life situations has been attributed to damage to these areas (Purdy, 2002). The fact that there is such differentiation in the literature highlights the fact that EF comprises a range of component sub-processes. However, most of the research on EF and aphasia has examined isolated aspects of EF and the need for composite profiling exists. As Purdy (2002, p. 557) has argued:

> studies should strive to operationally define the sub-processes of executive functioning and their interrelationships. Studies should also attempt to determine the relationship between executive function skills and communication. This understanding will ultimately lead to more appropriate and efficient management of clients.

One framework that we have found useful is Barkley's model (1997), which highlights four components of EF. This theory postulates that the critical units of EF that provide the opportunity for and protect self-regulating activities are behavioural inhibition and interference control. The EFs themselves comprise working memory, internalisation of speech (planning, problem solving), reconstitution (fluency, creativity, analysis and synthesis of behaviour), and regulation of affect (emotional self-control, regulation of drive and motivation). Details of this theory in application to aphasia may be found in Frankel and Penn (2007). As Hartley has done in the field of traumatic brain injury (Hartley, 1995), we have highlighted the proposed manifestation of EFs in conversation using this framework in Table 1.

Assessment of EF and its subcomponents in aphasia is challenging and is compounded by a number of variables. A feature of measurement is that testing simpler cognitive skills does not highlight EF deficits or advantages. More complex tasks are required (Bialystok et al., 2005; Butler, Rorsman, Hill, & Tuma, 1993; Godefroy & Rousseaux, 1997; Stuss, 1993) and for individuals with aphasia there is a need to administer control tasks in addition to executive tasks to rule out confounding variables such as neglect. Many tests have a verbal bias and pose challenges to the understanding of their novel requirements (Keil & Kaszniak, 2002). Tests often rely on the amount of time taken to complete the test, and modifications are necessary to accommodate impaired processing or motoric function (Frankel, Penn, & Ormond-Brown, 2007). Consequently, several studies have found that people with aphasia perform significantly worse on tests of verbal intelligence, memory (Kertesz & McCabe, 1975), and spatial and conceptual abilities (Hamsher, 1998) than non-brain-injured individuals or persons with right hemisphere (RH) brain damage.

Current research suggests that bilingual speakers have a different kind of readiness (Abutalebi & Green, 2007) with enhanced attentional control or a cognitive reserve. Further, these processes appear to extend into ageing (Bialystok, 2007). This leads to the possibility that the bilingual brain is more resistant to the influence of brain damage after a stroke. If, as Abutalebi and Green (2007, p. 247) suggest, "inhibition is a key mechanism in language control", it follows that measurement of inhibition will help explain some of the compensatory behaviours we see in the language/s of the bilingual individual with aphasia. Testing this hypothesis requires the development of a suitable EF battery. The challenge to the researcher is in the design of an appropriate EF battery that at the same time bypasses the confounding variables in aphasia yet is complex enough for EF advantages to emerge.

In prior research we reported on the development of an EF battery for aphasia based on the Barkley framework and taking into account the methodological challenges described above (Frankel et al., 2007). Here we examine the performance on this battery of two bilingual and eight monolingual individuals with aphasia and see whether conversational behaviours suggest an interface with that cognitive profile. The fact that conversation represents a complex integration of processes that requires planning, sequencing, organisation, and monitoring during novel activity makes it the ideal communicative vehicle through which to observe breakdown or preservation of complex EF and cognitive functioning (Penn, 2000; Rende, 2000).

The aim of this study is to examine whether the performance of bilingual persons on a specially devised EF battery is different from that of monolingual participants. Further, we examined the conversational output of the participants, based on the assumption that conversation—by definition a complex task—would provide a window onto the application of these processes.

METHOD

We investigated the EF profiles of individuals who had suffered a stroke to determine whether the profiles of participants with bilingual or multilingual

TABLE 1
Executive functions and discourse features corresponding to intact or impaired function based on Barkley's model (1997)

Executive function	Definition	Proposed manifestation
Behavioural Inhibition		
Response inhibition	The ability to inhibit a prepotent[*] response to an event and stop an ongoing response, which thereby permits a delay in the decision to respond.	**Intact** • The ability to recognise and stop ineffective communication strategies. **Deficit** • Perseveration.
Interference control	The protection of the period of delay from disruption by competing events and responses.	**Intact** • The ability to remain committed to behavioural chains or goal directed behaviours such as pursuing a repair trajectory or sustaining a topic of conversation without distraction. **Deficit** • Interruptions. • Abrupt topic changes with no or little relation to previous topic. • Difficulty staying on topic, tangential output.
Working memory	The ability to hold events in mind and manipulate or act on these events. Also included are retrospective and prospective functions—the ability to reach into the past and recall or anticipate future outcomes. Cross temporal organisation of behaviour.	**Intact** • The ability to recall what was said, integrate it with current conversation and anticipate how future actions will impact on conversational success. • Adaptation of previously stated information in different ways to continue or clarify communication. • The ability to grasp and communicate a sense of time. • The ability to organise behaviour across a temporal delay. **Deficit** • Difficulty linking previously stated information to current context. • Notably few or absent references to past or future events. • Inability or decreased ability to maintain coherent sense of events or topic.
Planning/Problem solving	The ability to produce rule-governed behaviour, engage in description and reflection, and generation of rules and meta-rules.	**Intact** • The ability to describe and reflect on communicative behaviour. • The ability to engage in problem solving to effect repair by the selection and utilisation of alternative strategies to drive successful communication. **Deficit** • Inability or decreased ability to engage in self reflection regarding communication. • Inability or decreased ability to plan discourse resulting in confabulation, rambling or incoherent output.

TABLE 1
Continued

Executive function	Definition	Proposed manifestation
Reconstitution	Analysis and synthesis of behaviour, verbal and behavioural fluency, creativity and behavioural simulations.	**Intact** • The ability to generate and have available a number of communication strategies for adaptive and flexible use. • Creativity in the use of communication strategies. **Deficit** • Decreased ability to generate alternate communication strategies. • Decreased verbal output in terms of amount of words or number of ideas.

*The prepotent response is defined as that response for which immediate reinforcement (positive or negative) is available or has previously been associated with that response.

backgrounds differed from those of monolinguals. In addition, we investigated the manifestation of these EF profiles in discourse, particularly in conversation. Data came from a larger corpus obtained during a research study (Frankel, 2008) correlating the EF profiles of these individuals with conversation. Participants were required to undergo a battery of executive tests in order to obtain baseline measures for the original study and were also recorded for 30 minutes while conversing with a familiar interlocutor. Conversations were recorded at least four different times over the course of the initial study and these transcripts were used for the current investigation.

Participants

Two female participants with bilingual/multilingual backgrounds, GB and TD, as well as eight other individuals who had experienced a stroke were recruited for the study. The bilingual participants and seven of the monolingual participants had aphasia as a result of a single acquired focal injury to the brain. Two participants (JR and FG) had a RH lesion, but JR (who was left-handed) displayed frank aphasia on the Western Aphasia Battery (WAB) whereas FG had a profile characteristic of right hemisphere syndrome. In order to control for possible confounding variables (e.g., apraxia, neglect, depression), precautions were taken with selection criteria. Neurological assessments and examinations were available to the consulting neurologist to confirm diagnosis. All participants had successful completion of secondary education (12 years) and were fluent in English. All participants were in the chronic stages of recovery and had no visual or hearing impairments. Importantly they had to demonstrate an ability to comply with the EF test demands and persons with severe language difficulties (as measured on the WAB) were thus excluded. Pertinent participant details are provided in Table 2. The details of the two participants with bilingual backgrounds are highlighted in bold. Both bilingual participants have used English predominantly for many years. Statistical analysis revealed no difference in severity scores on WAB (tested in English) between bilingual and monolingual participants $t(8) = 0.023$ ns.

TABLE 2
Participant details

Participant	Age	Gender	Site of lesion	Type of aphasia	WAB Aphasia Quotient	Language background	Time since onset (years)	Education	Previous occupation
GB (Bilingual)	**57**	F	**Left fronto-parietal cortex**	**Conduction**	**75**	**English/Afrikaans**	**6**	**16 years**	**Administrative manager for old age home**
TD (Multilingual)	**54**	F	**Left tempero-parietal cortex**	**Anomic**	**72.8**	**Tswana, Zulu, Shangaan, Xhosa, English, Afrikaans, Sotho, French, Russian**	**17**	**12 + interrupted tertiary education**	**Poet, Political activist**
CS	67	M	Left postero-inferior parietal cortex	Anomic	86	English	3	15 years	Previously and currently – Car salesman
FG	67	F	Right tempero-parietal cortex	Right hemisphere syndrome	98.4	English	5	18 years	Nurse
JD	60	F	Left fronto-parietal cortex	Conduction	65.9	English	5	15 years	Mechanic
JH	40	M	Left fronto-parietal cortex	Broca's	78.1	English	8	18+ years	Architect
JR	53	F	Right fronto-temporal cortex (left handed)	Conduction	88	English	6	13 years	PA for corporate managing director
MZ	64	F	Left postero-parietal cortex	Conduction	79.8	English	3	14 years	Book keeper
MS	59	F	Left fronto-parietal cortex	Anomic	93.4	English	5	18+ years	Art and Language teacher
PF	63	M	Left fronto-parietal lobe	Broca's	31.3	English	1	16 years	Import manager for mining company

Procedure

Participants were tested on an executive test battery designed to tap critical areas of EF in line with Barkley's (1997) model of behavioural inhibition and executive functions. This battery has been developed to bypass the cognitive, motoric, and linguistic limitations imposed on the participants by the presence of aphasia. Details regarding the theory, construction and application of this EF battery are provided in Frankel and Penn (2007). Table 3 summarises the constructs under investigation and the tests used to compile the relevant battery for this research.

Clearance for the larger study was obtained through the Committee for Research on Human Subjects at the University of the Witwatersrand. Potential recruits participated in an interview in their home environments with family members present when requested. Verbal and written consent was obtained after an interactive explanation of the study, supported with modified materials for those with aphasia. A waiting period of up to a month was provided to give participants an opportunity to make a decision and consult with significant others should they wish to do so.

Tests were administered in the participants' homes under optimal conditions. The battery took approximately 1½ hours to administer, although some participants required more time. Testing breaks were taken whenever requested and at the tester's discretion. Performance was scored and tables drawn up to indicate areas of preserved and deficient functioning for each of the constructs assessed. Due to the small sample size, non-parametric statistics were used to rank performance (Mann-Whitney U test; Siegel, 1956).

Conversations were recorded in accordance with guidelines presented by Ten Have (1999) in relation to capturing naturally occurring conversations. Family members, friends, or the second author (when needed) served as the participants' interlocutors. In the case of the bilingual participants, the interlocutors were

TABLE 3
Constructs and test battery for assessing EF

Construct	Test
Behavioural inhibition	
1. Interference control	1. Stroop Color Word Test (Golden, 1978)
2. Inhibition	2. Trail Making Test (Lezak, Howieson & Loring, 2004)
Working memory	1. Self Ordered Pointing Test (Spreen & Strauss, 1998)
	2. Complex Figures (Spreen & Strauss, 1998)
	3. Wisconsin Card Sorting Test (Ormond Software Enterprises, 1999)[*]
Internalisation of speech	1. Tower of London (Shallice, 1982)
Planning/Problem solving	2. Raven's Progressive Matrices (Raven, Raven, & Court, 1998)
Reconstitution	1. Five Point Test (Spreen & Strauss, 1998)
	2. Design Fluency (Spreen & Strauss, 1998)

*The categorisation of the WCST as a working memory test is worth noting. Traditionally the WCST is the classic test of set shifting, however it is also characterised as a test of working memory owing to its assessment of effective processing of feedback information to monitor and adjust performance (Barkley, 1998). The close link between inhibition and working memory functions also leads Barkley (1997) to conclude that some functions like set shifting in the face of a prescribed set of sub-goals are dependent on working memory functions.

bilingual. Transcripts were prepared for each of 40 separate interactions (4 per participant). These transcripts were then distributed to four raters, three of whom were blind to the bilingual status of the participants. Following the guidelines of Barbour (2001), a process of multiple coding strategies was used in order to ensure rigour and derive consensus. The samples of each participant were scrutinised independently by each of the four raters in order to characterise the features of the conversation and the presence or absence of executive characteristics as outlined in Table 1, using the framework of Conversation Analysis. The judges reached independent conclusions regarding the presence of executive features within the conversations of bilingual and monolingual speakers and these analyses were then compared. A table was drawn up for each of the 10 participants noting the presence or absence of executive features of their conversation.

RESULTS

Table 4 and Table 5 present the results of the study using the EF battery and the analysis of conversation respectively. In Table 4 the scores on the battery are presented in relation to established norms.

As can be seen from Table 4, the executive profiles of the two bilingual aphasia participants in this study are remarkably different from those of the monolingual ones. There is a significant difference between the scores of the bilingual participants (GB and TD) and those of the monolingual participants according to the Mann Whitney U test on the Stroop Colour Word Test $p < .10$; Trail Making Test $p < .05$; Self-ordered Pointing test $p < .05$; Complex Figures Test $p < .10$; Wisconsin Card Sorting Test $p < .05$; Tower of London $p < .05$; Raven's Progressive Matrices $p < .05$; Five Point Test $p < .05$; and Design Fluency $p < .05$. Except for the performance on the Raven's Progressive Matrices, on which all participants scored below the norm on measures of behavioural inhibition, working memory, planning and problem solving, and reconstitution (cf. Bailey et al., 1981; Kertesz & McCabe, 1975), the bilingual participants' scores were within normal limits and were significantly different from the group as a whole. Inspection of Table 4 also demonstrates the wide variety in performance between participants in the study, despite the selection criteria that matched severity and almost equivalent scores on the WAB aphasia quotient in some cases (see Table 2).

Of interest too is the performance of the patient with right hemisphere damage (FG) whose EF seems particularly and uniformly compromised, and lends support to the cluster of executive deficits in this syndrome described by Myers (1999) and also to the potential strength of the battery in differentiating different aetiologies.

The strong and unexpected finding of a differentiation between the bilingual and monolingual participants on these neuropsychological tests shows that language history may indeed be a profoundly influential variable in participant selection for research studies of individuals with aphasia (Roberts, Code, & McNeil, 2003), affecting language performance beyond the level of the structured language test. Although there were only two bilingual participants in the present study, the effects reported here support the neuropsychological and neuroimaging evidence showing that there is something different about bilingual participants. The EF battery seemed very sensitive to these differences. Further, the results suggest that these differences are due to better inhibitory control, increased flexibility, better working memory and planning, heightened resistance to interruption, and evidence of creativity and

TABLE 4
Performance of bilingual versus monolingual participants on EF test battery

Construct	Norms	Bilinguals		Monolinguals								Group mean
		GB	TD	CS	FG	JD	JH	JR	MZ	MS	PF	
Behavioural Inhibition												
Stroop Color Word Test*	Ratio of colour-word errors to colour errors Mean: 2.28 (.70)	1.14	1.64	30	64	1.6	5.63	3.5	32	4.13	1	17.7325
Trail Making Test**	Ratio of time to completion of Trail B to Trail A Mean: 2.21	2.15	1.26	3.47	2.6	2.55	2.74	3.78	3.7	4.69	1.47	3.125
Working Memory												
Self-Ordered Pointing Test**	Number of errors Means: 4.68 (2.53)	2	4	13	19	15	24	26	20	20	20	19.625
Complex Figures*	Raw score Mean: 14.88 (6.95)	22	17	6.5	14	10	7	0	7.5	18.5	17.5	10.125
Wisconsin Card Sorting Test**	Total category sorts Norm: 4–6	4	4	3	1	7	0	3	1	1	1	2.125
Internalisation of Speech/Planning/Problem Solving												
Tower of London**	Standard score SS: 85–115	95	125	65	0	0	0	0	0	0	0	8.125
Raven's Progressive Matrices**	Percentile rank Percentile rank: ≥45	41	10	12	0	13	9	4	4	6	9	7.125
Reconstitution												
Five Point Test**	Cut off point ≤15% perseveration	0	5	20	50	14.7	22.5	25	30	47	17.5	28.3375
Design Fluency**	Number of unique designs Mean: 15.5	16	15	3	2	3	5	4	4	4	8	4.125

Grey areas reflect below average score.
*Significant difference between bilingual and monolingual group at $p < .10$ level.
**Significance at $p < .05$ level.

TABLE 5
Presence/absence of executive features in conversational samples of 10 stroke patients

Participant	Response inhibition	Interference control	Working memory	Internalisation of speech	Reconstitution	Conversational characteristics
GB (Bilingual)	√	√	√	√	√	Intact turn taking, topic management, and repair.
TD (Bilingual)	√	√	√	√	√	Intact turn taking, topic management, and repair.
CS	X	X	√	√	I	Turn taking impaired by extended length and interruptions; topic management impaired by fragmented shifts and poor topic maintenance; repair impaired by failure to respond to requests for clarification.
FG	X	X	X	X	√	Turn taking impaired by extended length and interruptions; topic management impaired by tangentiality and failure to initiate; repair intact.
JD	√	√	√	X	X	Intact turn taking; topic management mostly intact with attempts at initiation and shift; repair impaired by limited strategy use and reliance on interlocutor.
JH	X	I	X	X	X	Turn taking impaired by delayed response, reduced length and content; topic management impaired by lack of initiation and limited contribution to shift; repair impaired by lack of initiation attempts and total reliance on interlocutor.
JR	X	X	X	X	√	Intact turn taking; topic management impaired by poor organisation and incoherence; repair intact.
MZ	X	X	X	X	√	Turn taking impaired by extended length; topic management impaired by lack of organisation, incoherence, irrelevance and tangentiality; repair intact.
MS	X	I	I	X	X	Intact turn taking; topic management mostly intact with some topic perseveration; repair impaired by perseveration and limited strategy use.

TABLE 5
Continued

Participant	Response inhibition	Interference control	Working memory	Internalisation of speech	Reconstitution	Conversational characteristics
PF	I	I	I	I	I	Turn taking function intact, but cannot utilise turn space effectively; topic management completely impaired; repair impaired by perseveration and lack of strategy use despite multiple attempts at revision.

$\sqrt{}$ = Feature is clearly evident to all judges across transcripts. X = Feature is clearly deficient to all judges across transcripts. I = There is no clear pattern of strength or deficit observed; variable or inconsistent presentation across transcripts, or lack of consensus among raters.

flexibility, confirming the observations of Bialystok (2007) regarding cognitive control advantages of bilingual participants.

We explored these advantages more specifically in conversational transcripts of the participants to test the findings of prior research linking the identification of compensatory strategies in interaction (e.g., Penn, 2007; Ramsberger, 2005). While these strategies have a variety of linguistic forms, their origins do not appear to lie in the language profile alone but in the area of cognitive control. The conversational samples of all participants were therefore rated for the presence or absence of certain conversational features, as delineated in Table 1. These results are summarised in Table 5. In line with Stemler's (2004) suggestions, clear agreements between raters are reflected. Percentage agreement was calculated to be 82%.

Inspection of Table 5 suggests the presence of strong conversational strategies in the bilingual participants who showed preserved topic control and initiation, repair, and conversational flexibility. While some of these strategies were present in transcripts of the monolingual persons, their profiles seemed scattered or inconsistent, correlating with EF profiles and manifesting in specific conversational disruptions such as poor topic control, perseveration, lack of repair, and digression.

Some examples from the transcripts are provided in Appendix A, illustrating executive features in conversation and narrative discourse by the two bilingual participants as well as recorded discourse from bilingual speakers with aphasia from a data corpus collected by Penn, Venter, and Ogilvy (2001). The results suggest that some of the shifting strategies in the bilingual individuals may be linked to their profile of cognitive flexibility. We could ask whether factors other than EF explain the differential performance of the two bilingual participants on this test battery. However, these differences cannot be attributed to age, type and severity of aphasia, or educational background. There may be lesion differences but unfortunately we do not have the benefit of advanced neuroimaging for the participants. However, information about site of lesion (available from their neurology reports and CT scans) suggests no marked differences between the lesions of the bilingual and monolingual participants with aphasia, and reinforces the view that EF has wide neurological representation. Given the widely dispersed nature of EF (Green, 2005), the fact that the monolingual patients without overt frontal damage are still having difficulty on the EF battery and conversational tasks is not unexpected. Clearly, explanations about the exclusive role of the frontal areas in EF are oversimplified.

A detailed analysis of the monolingual performance is beyond the scope of this paper. However, the performance of participant MS is described in detail in a recent report and demonstrates her marked conversational breakdown characterised by inflexibility and perseveration (Frankel et al., 2007). There is a marked similarity of her lesion (and aphasia type and severity) to the bilingual participant GB. Yet GB shows a clear ability to sustain a conversation over time. GB demonstrates intact turn-taking skills, taking her turn promptly at appropriate transitional spaces. Her contributions show her to be clearly engaged with the topic under discussion, and she is further able to initiate and shift topics as well as respond to topic termination. She independently initiates and engages a number of repair strategies with success. GB's anomia, although significant, does not interfere with her ability to hold a conversation and she tolerates interruptions well. Thus, in marked contrast to MS, GB benefits from supportive scaffolding provided by her interlocutor in the interactions recorded and she appears to hold her own in terms of conversational flow. As in the case of the individuals with aphasia described by Ramsberger (2005), the different EF profiles of GB and MS seem to account for these differences.

TD also demonstrated an ability to participate in conversation. She takes turns in both the single and the collaborative floor, although her participation in the latter is reduced. She clearly follows topics and contributes appropriately to shift and termination as well as being able to introduce lines of discussion herself. Again, this ability is more evident when talking to one interlocutor than in collaboration. She shows the ability to self-repair and her conversation flows. She is able to use external cues, facial expression, and gesture to supplement her communication.

Again the impact of RH damage on conversational features was highlighted in our analysis and reinforced the impact of this syndrome on aspects of discourse (Myers, 1999). The participant with RH syndrome (FG) showed markedly impaired conversational competence (including poor topic control and digression), attributable at least in part it would seem to her concomitant profile of impaired EF, including problems with behavioural inhibition, working memory, planning and problem solving, and reconstitution.

DISCUSSION

Our data, although preliminary, suggest that some of the characteristics in the conversational output of our bilingual participants with aphasia may be a reflection of compensatory strategies, which are linked to the integrity of EF. Their performance on an EF battery was significantly different from that of monolingual brain-damaged persons, and the differences in their conversational profiles could not be accounted for in terms of linguistic symptoms, aphasia type, and severity alone. Clearly, the application of both linguistic and cognitive processes is required for the steering of conversation. The emerging evidence in recent research indicates that there may be some cognitive control differences between bilingual and monolingual brains. This is borne out by our findings and suggests some fascinating future directions.

In our two bilingual cases, their language environments at the time of testing were primarily English and hence opportunities to use more than one language were limited. However, the advantages of flexibility that authors such as Bialystok (1999,

2007; Bialystok et al., 2005) suggest are characteristic of bilingual speakers, appear to be present and robust, and are reflected in their EF as well as, importantly, in the complex task of conversation. Our findings have many potential implications for therapy, particularly with the bilingual individual with aphasia. They may also help to resolve some of the inconsistencies in the literature pertaining to differential patterns of recovery of language in bilingual aphasia, choice of language for therapy, the relative response to therapy and the transfer of therapy in one language to the other language(s) of the bilingual individual with aphasia (see, for example, Meinzer, Obleser, Flaisch, Eulitz, & Rockstroh, 2007). For example, there has been some discrepancy in the literature as to which language should be used for therapy. Suggestions have been linked to the choice of one language over another. While some suggest that the patient's home language should be the language of choice for treatment, others believe that the most frequently used language, or the dominant language, or the language that appears spontaneously should be targeted. The possible interfering effect of using two languages has been commented on (Fabbro et al., 2000), although Kohnert and Derr (2004, p. 14) warn that clinicians often "look for reasons to discount one language in favour of the other" when choosing to provide language therapy in one language only. Marrero, Golden and Espe-Pfeifer (2002, pp. 474–475) believe that "therapy is best conducted in the stronger language in order to best tap internal cognitive processes", but they also suggest that therapy should be conducted in the language that "maximizes the client's understanding and insight".

The choice of monolingual or bilingual therapy is clearly a complex matter that should be individualised and depends heavily on context and environment. However, given the results of this study, there is support for the suggestion that EF has a role to play in this choice. Little attention has been given to the possible deliberate deployment of bilingual language therapy and an approach to intervention that is bilingual (e.g., Kohnert, 2004; Kohnert & Derr, 2004) seems to be reinforced by our findings. If EF seems to be well preserved, the compensatory and shifting strategies that the individual has applied premorbidly may be brought to bear after the stroke to facilitate interaction. It could be argued that if those control functions are the strength of the patient, then a bilingual approach to therapy may enhance pragmatic competence and offer a variety of choices especially if the language environment will support such flexibility. Clearly bilingual therapy in a monolingual environment will have little utility. However, in a context that promotes strategies such as code switching and linguistic shift, it might facilitate and enhance functional recovery. Indeed some such metalinguistic approaches to aphasia intervention (e.g., Holland & Penn, 1995; Penn & Beecham, 1992) have been found to be useful. It should be noted, however, that bilingual therapy may not be easy to implement in an individual with limited capacity on EF tasks, and this might strengthen an argument for monolingual language therapy in those cases.

Our hypothesis regarding the role of EF in conversation may account for another unresolved issue in the field regarding the relative transfer of therapy effects in one language to other languages. Several studies have claimed that the effects of therapy in one language usually transfer to the other non-targeted language(s) to some degree (Fredman, 1975). However, other studies have demonstrated no transfer of therapy effects (e.g., Meinzer et al., 2007), greater recovery in the targeted language (e.g., Gil & Goral, 2004; Watamori & Sasanuma, 1978), and/or only partial recovery in the untreated languages (e.g., Filiputti, Tavano, Vorano, De Luca, & Fabbro, 2002). Based on reported data in the literature, Gil and Goral (2004) conclude that treatment effects do transfer to the non-treated language to some extent, but that these effects may be small and may not transfer to all language modalities. They suggest that factors such as premorbid language function, usage, fluency, linguistic structure of the languages, as well as the type of therapy (Kohnert, 2004) have an impact on the amount of transfer that takes place. Patterns of generalisation and cross-linguistic transfer may depend on the method of learning, the nature of the treatment and the learning system that is activated during therapy (Galvez & Hinckley, 2003). In addition, the transfer effects observed in some studies may be due to spontaneous recovery processes rather than a genuine transfer of benefit (Gil & Goral, 2004).

We believe that the possibility of underlying cognitive processes as explanatory factors needs to be explored. While it is interesting that there is neurological evidence for differential recovery effects for treated and untreated languages (Abutalebi & Green, 2007; Green, 2005), therapy approaches are stimulating inhibition mechanisms of the recovering brain (rather than language processes per se) and hence are utilising control rather than language functions. We should certainly be more cautious about taking the language history of the patient, and recognise that aside from other influences that we normally control for, the language history may have a very important role to play in accounting for results. This role is not solely in the linguistic domain but extends to the cognitive and pragmatic domain. This reinforces the suggestion that the assessment of executive functions should possibly become a regular component of the clinical battery, particularly in determining the therapeutic approach to be used. It appears to provide a firm explanatory paradigm for clinical endeavour and apparently has potential to distinguish aetiologies, language backgrounds, and cognitive styles.

We are not suggesting, of course, that monolingual individuals with aphasia do not have the potential to use EF. As our own findings imply and the literature suggests, some such individuals perform well on EF tasks and are judged better communicators (Miyake et al., 2000). Our preliminary results suggest, however, that at least some bilingual patients may have enhanced EF bases to their language, potentially reinforced by their context and providing some additional immunity or protection from brain damage (as Bialystok, 2007, has hypothesised in the case of ageing). Put in another way, executive capacity enables the development of compensatory strategies that may have some unique manifestations in bilingual participants. The advantages of these compensatory strategies may not play out on standard language tasks, but will manifest in more taxing tasks such as conversation. As we have shown, many of the symptoms in our data pool of discourse appear to be reflections of underlying cognitive processes. The ability to initiate, sustain, return to a conversation, and assume responsibility for repair requires cognitive integrity. As Hartley (1995) has argued in the area of traumatic brain injury, the individual components of EF may play out in different ways in conversation. It would thus seem important to unpack the broad term EF into its component parts and clearly there is neuroimaging evidence for this claim (Abutalebi & Green, 2007). Recognition of these component parts allows for individualised profiling and hopefully individualised intervention.

In sum, when making treatment decisions, EF might explain differential recovery and response to therapy across all patient groups (Ramsberger, 2005). However this seems to be particularly true for the bilingual person and this might guide the therapist towards therapeutic choices, including selection of languages for therapy and development of compensatory strategies. Relatively intact EF might be an indication for bilingual therapy, provided this is supported by the language environment. In addition, where EFs are well preserved, we would aim to develop patient-centred compensatory strategies. These strategies could be conversational or could directly address one or more of the executive skills such as direct attention training (Coelho, 2005; Helm-Estabrooks et al., 2000; Ramsberger, 2005; Sohlberg & Mateer, 2001; Sohlberg, Johnson, Paule, Raskin, & Mateer, 2001; Sturm et al., 1997). In other cases, our focus may be better placed on providing a supportive context that will compensate for conversational and executive deficits. Indeed, this is the approach of some of the partner-focused therapies with a focus on conversation (e.g., Kagan, Black, Duchan, Simmons-Mackie, & Square, 2001). All of these possibilities require further examination. Clearly this topic is in its infancy and presents methodological and analytic challenges. There are obvious limitations to our preliminary work. The first is that because this was part of a larger study the bilingual patients were not tested in more than one of their languages, and this will be our future goal. Further, there is a need to supplement some of our conclusions with advanced neuroimaging and with some carefully controlled intervention studies. However, our findings raise some potentially important clinical implications both for monolingual and bilingual persons. We are therefore confident that the field of bilingualism is a profoundly fruitful domain for examining the interface between cognition, language, and context and will strengthen many future therapeutic endeavours.

REFERENCES

Abutalebi, J., & Green, D. (2007). Bilingual language production: The neurocognition of language representation and control. *Journal of Neurolinguistics, 20*, 242–275.

Bailey, S., Powell, G., & Clark, E. (1981). A note on intelligence and recovery from aphasia: The relationship between Raven's Matrices Scores and change on the Schuell Aphasia Test. *British Journal of Disorders of Communication, 16*, 193–203.

Barbour, R. (2001). Checklists for improving rigour in qualitative research: A case of the tail wagging the dog? *British Medical Journal, 322*, 1115–1117.

Barkley, R. (1997). Behavioural inhibition, sustained attention, and executive functions: Constructing a unifying theory of ADHD. *Psychological Bulletin, 121*, 65–94.

Beeke, S., Wilkinson, R., & Maxim, J. (2003a). Exploring aphasic grammar 1: A single case analysis of conversation. *Clinical Linguistics and Phonetics, 17*, 81–107.

Beeke, S., Wilkinson, R., & Maxim, J. (2003b). Exploring aphasic grammar 2: Do language testing and conversation tell a similar story? *Clinical Linguistics and Phonetics, 17*, 109–134.

Bialystok, E. (1999). Cognitive complexity and attentional control in the bilingual mind. *Child Development, 70*, 636–644.

Bialystok, E. (2007). Cognitive effects of bilingualism: How linguistic experience leads to cognitive change. *The International Journal of Bilingual Education and Bilingualism, 10*, 210–223.

Bialystok, E., Craik, F., Grady, C., Chau, W., & Ishii, R. (2005). Effect of bilingualism on cognitive control in the Simon task: Evidence from MEG. *NeuroImage, 24*, 40–49.

Butler, R., Rorsman, I., Hill, J., & Tuma, R. (1993). The effects of frontal brain impairment on fluency: Simple and complex paradigms. *Neuropsychology, 7*, 519–529.

Coelho, C. (2005). Direct attention training as a treatment for reading impairment in mild aphasia. *Aphasiology, 19*, 275–283.

Crinion, J., Turner, R., Grogan, A., Hanakawa, T., Noppeney, U., & Devlin, J., et al. (2006). Language control in the bilingual brain. *Science, 312*, 1537–1540.

Crosson, B., Moore, A., Gopinath, K., White, K., Wierenga, C., & Gaiefsky, M., et al. (2005). Role of the right and left hemispheres in recovery of function during treatment of intention in aphasia. *Journal of Cognitive Neuroscience, 17*, 392–406.

Fabbro, F., Skrap, M., & Aglioti, S. (2000). Pathological switching between languages following frontal lesions in a bilingual patient. *Journal of Neurology, Neurosurgery and Psychiatry, 68*, 650–652.

Filiputti, D., Tavano, A., Vorano, L., De Luca, G., & Fabbro, F. (2002). Nonparallel recovery of languages in a quadrilingual aphasic patient. *International Journal of Bilingualism, 6*, 395–410.

Frankel, T. (2008). *Conversation intelligence after stroke: A drug trial.* Unpublished doctoral dissertation, University of the Witwatersrand, Johannesburg, South Africa.

Frankel, T., & Penn, C. (2007). Perseveration and conversation in TBI: Response to pharmacological intervention. *Aphasiology, 21*, 1039–1078.

Frankel, T., Penn, C., & Ormond-Brown, D. (2007). Executive dysfunction as an explanatory basis for conversation symptoms of aphasia: A pilot study. *Aphasiology, 21*, 814–828.

Fredman, M. (1975). The effect of therapy given in Hebrew on the home language of the bilingual or polyglot adult aphasic in Israel. *International Journal of Communication Disorders, 10*, 61–19.

Galvez, A., & Hinckley, J. (2003). Transfer patterns of naming treatment in a case of bilingual aphasia. *Brain and Language, 87*, 173–174.

Gil, M., & Goral, M. (2004). Nonparallel recovery in bilingual aphasia: Effects of language choice, language proficiency, and treatment. *International Journal of Bilingualism, 8*, 191–219.

Godefroy, O., & Rousseaux, M. (1997). Novel decision making in patients with prefrontal or posterior brain damage. *Neurology, 49*, 695–701.

Golden, J. (1978). *Stroop Color and Word Test.* Illinois: Stoelting Company.

Goral, M., Levy, E., Obler, L., & Cohen, E. (2006). Cross-language lexical connections in the mental lexicon: Evidence from a case of trilingual aphasia. *Brain and Language, 98*, 235–247.

Green, D. (2005). The neurocognition of recovery patterns in bilingual aphasics. In J. Kroll & A. de Groot (Eds.), *Handbook of bilingualism: Psycholinguistic perspectives* (pp. 516–530). Oxford, UK: Oxford University Press.

Hartley, L. (1995). *Cognitive-communicative abilities following brain injury.* New York: Thomson Delmar Learning.

Hamsher, K. (1998). Intelligence and aphasia. In M. Sarno (Ed.), *Acquired aphasia* (pp. 339–372). New York: Academic Press.

Helm-Estabrooks, N., Tabor Connor, L., & Albert, M. (2000). Treating attention to improve auditory comprehension in aphasia. *Brain and Language, 74*, 469–472.

Holland, A., & Penn, C. (1995). Inventing therapy for aphasia. In L. Menn, M. O'Connor, K. Obler, & A. Holland (Eds.), *Non fluent aphasia in a multilingual world* (pp. 144–155). Amsterdam: Benjamins.

Jefferson, G. (2004). Glossary of transcript symbols with an Introduction. In G. Lerner (Ed.), *Conversation analysis: Studies from the first generation* (pp. 13–23). Philadelphia: John Benjamins.

Kagan, A., Black, S., Duchan, J., Simmons-Mackie, N., & Square, P. (2001). Training volunteers and conversation partners using "Supported Conversation for adults with Aphasia" (SCA). *Journal of Speech, Language, and Hearing Research, 44*, 624–638.

Keil, K., & Kaszniak, A. (2002). Examining executive function in individuals with brain injury: A review. *Aphasiology, 16*, 305–335.

Kertesz, A., & McCabe, P. (1975). Intelligence and aphasia: Performance of aphasics on Raven's Coloured Progressive Matrices (RCPM). *Brain and Language, 2*, 387–395.

Kohnert, K. (2004). Cognitive and cognate-based treatments for bilingual aphasia: A case study. *Brain and Language, 91*, 294–302.

Kohnert, K., & Derr, A. (2004). Language intervention with bilingual children. In B. Goldstein (Ed.), *Bilingual language development and disorders in Spanish–English speakers* (pp. 315–343). Baltimore: Brookes.

Korda, R., & Douglas, J. (1997). Attention deficits in stroke patients with aphasia. *Journal of Clinical and Experimental Neuropsychology, 19*, 525–542.

Lezak, M., Howieson, D., & Loring, D. (2004). *Neuropsychological assessment* (4th ed.). New York: Oxford University Press.

Lindfield, K., Polzik, D., & Roberts, J. (2000). Strategies underlying category free recall in anterior versus posterior aphasia. *Brain and Language, 74*, 498–501.

Marrero, M., Golden, C., & Espe-Pfeifer, P. (2002). Bilingualism, brain injury, and recovery: Implications for understanding the bilingual and for therapy. *Clinical Psychology Review, 22*, 463–478.

McNeil, M., Doyle, P., Hula, W., Rubinsky, H., Fossett, T., & Matthews, C. (2004). Using resource allocation theory and dual-task methods to increase the sensitivity of assessment in aphasia. *Aphasiology, 18*, 521–542.

Meinzer, M., Obleser, J., Flaisch, T., Eulitz, C., & Rockstroh, B. (2007). Recovery from aphasia as a function of language therapy in an early bilingual patient demonstrated by fMRI. *Neuropsychologia, 45*, 1247–1256.

Miyake, A., Emerson, M., & Friedman, N. (2000). Assessment of executive functions in clinical settings: Problems and recommendations. *Seminars in Speech and Language, 21*, 169–183.

Murray, L. (2000). The effects of varying attentional demands on the word-retrieval skills of adults with aphasia, right hemisphere brain-damage or no brain-damage. *Brain and Language, 72*, 40–72.

Murray, L., Holland, A., & Beeson, P. (1998). Spoken language of individuals with mild fluent aphasia under focused and divided-attention conditions. *Journal of Speech, Language, and Hearing Research, 41*, 213–227.

Myers, P. (1999). *Right hemisphere damage*. San Diego, CA: Singular.

Ogilvy, D., von Bentheim, I., Venter, A., Ulatowska, H., & Penn, C. (2000). Discourse, dialect and aphasia in the Western Cape. *South African Journal of Communication Disorders, 47*, 111–118.

Ormond Software Enterprises. (1999). *The Wisconsin Card Sorting Test*. Johannesburg: Digby Brown Enterprises.

Owen, A., Downes, J., Sahakian, B., Polkey, C., & Robbins, K. (1990). Planning and spatial working memory following frontal lobe lesions in man. *Neuropsychologia, 28*, 1021–1034.

Penn, C. (2000). Paying attention to conversation. *Brain and Language, 71*, 185–189.

Penn, C. (2007). Cultural dimensions of aphasia: Adding diversity and flexibility to the equation. In M. Ball & J. Damico (Eds.), *Clinical aphasiology: Future directions* (pp. 221–244). Hove, UK: Psychology Press.

Penn, C., & Beecham, R. (1992). Discourse therapy in multilingual aphasia: A case study. *Clinical Linguistics & Phonetics, 6*, 11–25.

Penn, C., Venter, A., & Ogilvy, D. (2001). Aphasia in Afrikaans: A preliminary analysis. *Journal of Neurolinguistics, 14*, 111–132.

Purdy, M. (1992). *The relationship between executive functioning ability and communicative success in aphasic adults*. Unpublished Doctoral dissertation, University of Connecticut.

Purdy, M. (2002). Executive function ability in persons with aphasia. *Aphasiology, 16*, 549–557.

Ramsberger, G. (2005). Achieving conversational success in aphasia by focusing on non-linguistic cognitive skills: A potentially promising new approach. *Aphasiology, 19*, 1066–1073.

Raven, J., Raven, J., & Court, J. (1998). *Standard Progressive Matrices*. Oxford, UK: Oxford Psychologists Press.

Rende, B. (2000). Cognitive flexibility: Theory and treatment. *Seminars in Speech and Language, 21*, 121–133.

Roberts, P., Code, C., & McNeil, M. (2003). Describing participants in aphasia research: Part 1. Audit of current practice. *Aphasiology, 17*, 911–932.

Shallice, T. (1982). Specific impairments of planning. *Philosophical Transactions of the Royal Society of London, 298*, 199–209.

Siegel, S. (1956). *Nonparametric statistics for the behavioural sciences*. Tokyo: McGraw Hill.

Sohlberg, M., Johnson, L., Paule, L., Raskin, S., & Mateer, C. (2001). *Attention Process Training-II (APT-II)*. Wake Forest, NC: Lash & Associates Publishing/Training Inc.

Sohlberg, M., & Mateer, C. (2001). Improving attention and managing attentional problems: Adapting rehabilitation techniques to adults with ADD. *Annals of the New York Academy of Sciences, 931*, 359–375.

Spreen, O., & Strauss, E. (1998). *A compendium of neuropsychological tests: Administration, norms and commentary* (2nd ed.). New York: Oxford University Press.

Stemler, S. (2004). A comparison of consensus, consistency, and measurement approaches to estimating inter-rater reliability. *Practical Assessment, Research and Evaluation, 9*(4). Retrieved 14 March 2008 from http://pareonline.net/getvn.asp?v=9&n=4.

Sturm, W., Willmes, K., Orgass, B., & Hartje, W. (1997). Do specific attention deficits need specific training? *Neuropsychological Rehabilitation, 7*, 81–103.

Stuss, D. (1993). Assessment of neuropsychological dysfunction in frontal lobe degeneration. *Dementia, 3–4*, 220–225.

Ten Have, P. (1999). *Doing conversation analysis*. London: Sage Publications.

Villiard, P. (1990). Agrammatism as evidence for a unified theory of word, phrase and sentence formation processes. In J-L. Nespoulous & P. Villiard (Eds.), *Morphology, phonology, and aphasia* (pp. 185–192). Berlin: Springer-Verlag.

Watamori, T., & Sasanuma, S. (1978). The recovery processes of two English–Japanese bilingual aphasics. *Brain and Language, 6*, 127–140.

APPENDIX A

Examples of executive functions as manifested in discourse of bilingual people with aphasia

Executive function			Example from discourse
Behavioural	009	R	oh and then has your sister gone back to Pretoria
Inhibition	010	TD	no ehm ((gets up to get a photo)) my brother this one
Response	011	R	oh
inhibition	012	TD	my brother this one B****
	013	R	oh oh
	014	TD	and then my suster Sh*** eh eh Rustenburg
Interference	212	MD	but what about alcohol? I never thought you guys drink alcohol.
control	213	R	little. well (.) not excessively
	214	MD	HEH?
	215	TD	ja
	216	R	not not (.) excessively but people
	217	MD	Ja but ordinary people we people drink
	218	**TD**	**Bible remember eh eh eh um (3) em**
	219	MD	((unintelligible))
	220	TD	<u>mm</u> mm mm ↓ mm mm ↓ Bible eh same thing wine
	221	MD	oh in the scriptures
	222	TD	Exactly so?
	223	MD	Ja well
	224	TD	Same thing
	225	MD	I never thought
	226	R	What?
	227	MD	because I know with Moslems very few of them drink
	228	TD	[Ja ja
	229	R	[ja
	230	MD	very few of them
	231	R	mm [but we have-]
	232	**TD**	**[But smoke]**
	233	R	smoke?
	234	TD	AAH! everybody
	235	R	ja
			[MD whistles]
	236	TD	and why? nobody knows.

Executive function	Example from discourse
Working memory (extract from data of Penn et al., 2001)	Okay, now I will tell you. You see, that time ((unintelligible)) counts back here to the 1940s. I think I was about sev seven or eight, around about time. I, what I used to do was, we used to beg for money and we, what I used to do is I is I was vvv at a young age, I was from the the age of four I was street wise. I knew everything about the streets in here in Cape Town where I mm and what we used to do was we go to the the eh eh eh umm station. I think I was about seven, ja about seven eight, it was jus, it was here just before the the King and Queen came here to South Africa. We used to beg there for money there and then one night the eh um a guy came to me and he said to me, wa wasn't only alo I wasn't alone, we was three or four to ah ah of the guys together. He asked to to to hand out pamphlets to people and eh I could deed, I could read but we were not, we just we were glad because the guy gave us a half a crown for for uh each to just to to to hand out the papers. And while we were handing out the papers the poll raid bay, the railway cops in the skay station they ca go go got hold of us and took us to to to to the jail which was eh eh eh in the old station was just outside of of the sssta station, it was wwwoodi (wooden) eyealalan a wood and iron jail. And this guys that, you must know, these guys were big ouens[1] and we are only small ah, we are only small pa ah pikkies[2] you know li (unintelligible). And he got hold of us and they started beating us and they wanted to know in Afrikaans "Who gave you these papers?" and ah I say "Well, a man gave us half a crown to hand out the papers." And he says "Well you're going to go to jail for a long long time." I've never ever forgotten that day because what he said to us afterwards. This was ANC[3] papers that we gave out. So we were just wwe were just (lambs) to get the we don't even know what it was to be about the ANC. That was in 1950, 1940 eh I think it was '47. Just as I said before, the Queen and King came and eh they told us to to eh's going to st lock us up. (Mr. C)

Planning/Problem solving

067	RB	but then why have you got her money if she's going to go to Wits
068	RB	or have I got the story all wrong again
069	GB	((to her son who is off camera)) please won't you uh uh look with my um file right next to my desk
070	GB	((talking to her husband again)) uh let's try again yesterday J*** wife is give me
071	RB	oh J*** wife gave you the money
072	GB	Yes
073	RB	Oh not the black lady
074	GB	No is the let's see oh thanks ((taking the file)) I hope it's in here
075	RB	You started speaking about J*** wife and then you started speaking about the black lady
076	GB	Ja oh alright ok here ((looking through the file))
077	RB	J*** H*** that's the the old man that's this one here
078	GB	Ja ja ja (.) there's
079	RB	T***
080	GB	T***
081	RB	Now Is that the that the one you're talking about?

Executive function		*Example from discourse*

Reconstitution

1. **Using external source to facilitate communication** – see example from Planning/Problem Solving above
2. **Using writing**

019	GB	Steps um
020	RB	Steps?
021	GB	[writes]
022	RB	sketches?

3. **Using circumlocution**

041	GB	did have the other one was uh (4) u:m (1) um (3) °jam° no um (3) uh that that little in the (1) fridge um
042	RB	Fishpaste?
043	GB	JA that I used that as well I did so it was well good

4. **Using gesture or enactment**

071	GB	sorry but anyhow it's I didn't hear that much but he swore that from (.) h-he got all this out again ↓ a- at the um (1)
072	RB	all the putty out
073	GB	ja uh:: (3) u:m (8)
074	RB	leg?
075	GB	NO sitting on your (acts out sitting and flushing) (.) TOILET ((hhh))
076	RB	((hhh)) oh on the toilet ok ja so all the putty he took out

5. **Breaking words up into component syllables to facilitate articulation**

043	GB	…all that everybody knitting except me ↑ I took my::: um (3) tap uh (1) tap [(.) es] (.) try
044	RB	[°try°]
045	RB	That's ↑ it.

[1] 'Ouens' is an Afrikaans word meaning *chap, fellow,* or *guy.*
[2] 'Pikkies' is an Afrikaans word meaning *little chap.*
[3] African National Congress.
MD is TD's husband.

APPENDIX B

Conversation analysis transcription symbols (Jefferson, 2004)

word	some form of stress, via pitch or amplitude
WORD	especially loud speech relative to surrounding talk
((laugh))	transcriber's descriptions, e.g., laughter or head nod
?	rising intonation
(.)	short pause
(0.0)	elapsed time in silence (in seconds)
(word)	especially dubious hearings or speaker identifications
°word°	softly spoken, quieter than the surrounding talk
[ ]	onset and offset of overlapping talk
:	prolongation of the immediately prior sound
-	cut-off
↑	shift into higher pitch in the utterance immediately following the arrow
↓	shift into lower pitch in the utterance immediately following the arrow
hhh	out breath or sigh
***	text omitted to protect participant's confidentiality
bold	bold is added to specific words, phrases or sentences for emphasis or to point out specific phenomena to the reader

APHASIOLOGY, 2010, 24 (2), 309–324

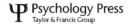

Model-driven intervention in bilingual aphasia: Evidence from a case of pathological language mixing

Ana Inés Ansaldo and Ladan Ghazi Saidi

Centre de recherche de l'Institut universitaire de gériatrie de Montréal, and University of Montreal, Quebec, Canada

Adelaida Ruiz

Facultad de Psicologia, Universidad de Buenos Aires, Argentina

Background: Speech-language pathologists are meeting an increasing number of bilingual clients. This poses a special challenge to clinical practice, given that bilingualism adds to the complexity of aphasia patterns and clinical decisions must be made accordingly. One question that has come to the attention of clinical aphasiologists is that of the language in which therapy should be administered. This issue becomes particularly relevant in cases of involuntary language switching, when choosing between L1 and L2 implies inhibiting one of the languages. Models of lexical selection in bilingual people offer a rationale for language choice based on the specificities of bilingual aphasia within each client.

Aims: To provide evidence for model-based intervention in bilingual aphasia, particularly in cases of pathological language switching.

Methods & Procedures: This paper reports a model-driven intervention in a case of involuntary language switching following aphasia in a Spanish–English bilingual client.

Outcomes & Results: Intervention tailored to the client's strengths resulted in improved communication skills thanks to the implementation of a self-regulated strategy to overcome involuntary language switching.

Conclusions: Model-driven descriptions of bilingual aphasia contribute to efficient intervention by identifying therapy approaches that take account of each client's language abilities. Further, clinical data analysed within models of bilingual language processing can provide evidence for dissociations between components of the bilingual lexical system.

Keywords: Bilingual aphasia; Intervention; Model-based; Pathological switching.

Given the demographic characteristics of the modern world, bilingualism is becoming the general rule, particularly in countries that receive a large number of immigrants. Further, in some countries, such as Canada and Belgium, bilingualism is a societal choice. The sociolinguistic dimensions of contemporary societies have an impact on clinical aphasiology. Consequently, there is a growing interest in intervention strategies and therapy efficacy with bilingual aphasia. When clients speak two or more languages a number of challenges related to their assessment and

Address correspondence to: Ana Inés Ansaldo, Centre de recherche de l'Institut universitaire de gériatrie de Montréal, 4565 Queen-Mary, Montreal, QC, Canada, H3W 1W5. E-mail: ana.ines.ansaldo@umontreal.ca

http://www.psypress.com/aphasiology   DOI: 10.1080/02687030902958423

intervention can arise, and this situation demands consideration in terms of the training given to future speech-language pathologists. Despite the increase in the number of bilingual clients, bilingual aphasia therapy has only recently become the focus of clinical aphasiology research. Hence, most of the studies published to date lack detailed descriptions of the nature of the deficits underlying the clinical signs observed, and do not provide a rationale for therapy choice. One of the main issues concerning intervention in bilingual aphasia concerns the choice of language for intervention. In this regard the literature is not extensive and there is no clear rationale to guide clinical decisions about treatment. Further, the extent to which therapy in one language transfers, or does not transfer, to the non-treated language remains a matter of debate.

BILINGUAL APHASIA THERAPY AND CROSS-LINGUISTIC EFFECTS

The concept of cross-linguistic transfer refers to the reciprocal influence that one language exerts on another. This question has most often been raised regarding lexical access, and has been studied mainly among healthy bilingual populations. Cross-linguistic transfer is considered to depend on cross-linguistic similarities, in addition to proficiency level (Ringbom, 2007). The study of cross-linguistic effects in healthy bilingual people has given rise to models of lexical access in bilingualism, some of which can account for experimental results obtained with a variety of paradigms (see Costa, Santesteban, & Caño, 2005, and Myers-Scotton, 2005, for an extensive discussion).

Data on the cross-linguistic effects of therapy in bilingual aphasia are relatively rare. Meinzer, Obleser, Flaisch, Eulitz, and Rockstroh (2007) examined the cross-linguistic effects of therapy in a patient's mother tongue (German) only. The participant was early bilingual with aphasia and naming deficits, and therapy consisted of a variety of games and shaping activities provided in a group setting. Meinzer et al. report improvement in the treated language only, concurrently with bilateral functional reorganisation, as evidenced by fMRI scanning during naming in German. Galvez and Hinckley (2003) administered therapy for naming deficits successively in both of the languages spoken by their patient. Therapy consisted of semantic and phonemic cueing, together with repetition tasks. Galvez and Hinckley reported beneficial effects after each training session for the treated language only, and no cross-linguistic transfer to the untreated language. Kohnert (2004) compared the effect of training on words with similar form and meaning across languages, called cognates, e.g., *rosa/rose*, with non-cognate words, e.g., *mesa/table*, in a 62-year-old Spanish–English bilingual patient with non-fluent aphasia, and observed cross-linguistic transfer effects from Spanish to English for cognate words only.

Some authors claim that the choice of language for therapy should be made on the basis of premorbid proficiency in the language. Edmonds and Kiran (2006) examined the effects of semantic treatment on naming in two unbalanced bilingual individuals with greater premorbid proficiency in one language than the other, and one balanced bilingual person with equal premorbid proficiency in both languages. The balanced bilingual patient showed improvement in both languages after therapy in L1, whereas the two unbalanced bilingual patients showed generalisation to the untreated language, when therapy was administered in L2, the less-proficient language. Edmonds and Kiran concluded that administering therapy in the less-dominant language might result in larger cross-linguistic effects for unbalanced bilingual patients.

Despite the interesting findings of these studies, the external validity of their results is limited by a number of methodological issues, particularly in terms of the rationale of therapy approach and language choice. Marrero, Golden, and Espe-Pfeifer (2002) argued that therapy choice requires an understanding of the individual client's profile. As in the case of aphasia therapy with monolingual clients, this may be rationally motivated by theories of bilingual language processing. In line with this perspective, Laganaro and Overton Venet (2001) developed a two-step computer-assisted remediation programme on the basis of an analysis of the deficits in a Spanish–English bilingual patient with alexia. Therapy was based on dual-route models of reading (Patterson, 1994), and administered successively in English and Spanish. The authors reported language-specific gains in tasks that address language-specific representations, and cross-linguistic effects when common processes were targeted. That study provides evidence of the utility of model-based descriptions to optimise intervention in bilingual aphasia.

This brief review of the literature shows there is still no definite answer about language choice in bilingual aphasia therapy. Most research has excluded one language and examined the extent of cross-linguistic transfer to the non-treated language. Historically, it has been assumed that bilingual aphasia therapy should be conducted in one language only, as therapy in both languages could favour inhibitory mechanisms and hinder full recovery (Hemphill, 1976; Lebrun, 1988). This may be a particular problem with patients who mix languages, where it has been argued that therapy should be limited to one language in order to avoid cross-language interference (Fabbro, 1999).

NEW PERSPECTIVES IN BILINGUAL APHASIA THERAPY

A different perspective on language choice in bilingual aphasia therapy stems from recent advances in the neurolinguistics of bilingualism. Green (2005) argues that, although methods used in monolingual interventions should work for bilingual patients, specific bilingual advantages should not be neglected when planning therapy. For example, Green argues that bilingual people with aphasia who show parallel recovery frequently self-cue and produce a correct word in the non-target language to retrieve the intended word. Therefore, depriving a bilingual patient of the use of preserved aspects of the non-treated language may not be justified (Ansaldo, Marcotte, Scherer, & Raboyeau, 2008). In our view, the preserved aspects of the bilingual language system should always be exploited to facilitate functional communication.

How should the language functioning of a bilingual patient be assessed? To determine the strengths and weaknesses of the language system, it is possible to describe a patient's deficit using psycholinguistic models of language processing in bilingual people. This approach can contribute to the development of therapy approaches by focusing on the roots of the impairment, rather than the surface signs. We will refer to this type of approach as model- or theory-driven intervention; it has also inspired much of the clinical research in aphasiology with monolingual people (Basso, 2003; Wertz, 1999). In bilingual aphasia, intervention has generally lacked a theory-driven rationale. However, when a theory-driven approach is used the results can be encouraging in terms of efficacy and efficiency of the intervention (Laganaro & Overton Venet, 2001).

In the present paper we report on a bilingual individual with word-finding difficulties. The most remarkable feature of performance was compulsory language switching within the context of conversations with monolingual partners. Although the client was aware of his language-switching deficit, switching could not be prevented even when he was explicitly asked to respond in one language. We provide a description of the language profile with reference to cognitive models of word production in bilingual people, and illustrate how this assessment led to the development of a therapy approach that was based specifically on preserved language abilities. We also show that this method resulted in improved communication, as well as a degree of cross-linguistic transfer of therapy benefits.

CASE DETAILS

EL is a right-handed, native Spanish-speaking bilingual man, who learnt some English during childhood. As an adult he completed graduate studies in English in the United States, where English became his everyday language. EL considered himself highly proficient in English. He spoke Spanish exclusively when he visited his hometown, but he continued to read books and newspapers in English. At the age of 56, EL suffered an embolic stroke that caused a lesion in the left internal capsule, including the left caudate nucleus. In the subacute phase after the stroke, EL showed transcortical mixed aphasia, with language mixing and language switching (Ansaldo & Marcotte 2007; Ruiz & Ansaldo, 1990). After receiving language therapy in Spanish for 8 months, he attained a plateau and was discharged from rehabilitation. EL was recruited for the present study 2 years after discharge.

EXPERIMENTAL INVESTIGATIONS

This study comprises three stages: a pre-therapy stage, a therapy stage, and a post-therapy stage. Measures of language performance were taken at the pre- and post-therapy stages, in both Spanish and English. In the pre-therapy stage EL's aphasia pattern was assessed, including picture-naming and translation skills, with nouns and verbs.

A control group of five Spanish–English bilingual individuals, matched on educational level, who had learnt English in adulthood and rated themselves as highly proficient in English, were tested on the same tasks. Following assessment, a model-based description of EL's performance on naming and translation tasks provided a rationale for language therapy. During the therapy stage of the study, EL received a model-based therapy approach, together with specific treatment for anomia. Therapy was provided in two 1-hour sessions per week. In the post-therapy stage, EL's aphasia pattern was reassessed, and he was tested on the naming and translation tasks again, with a list of treated words and a list of untreated words.

Pre-therapy stage

EL's aphasia patterns in Spanish and English were assessed separately, over a 3-day interval. On the first day of assessment, a monolingual speech-language pathologist

(SLP) assessed his performance in each language and sessions were recorded for later analysis. The aphasia pattern in Spanish was assessed first. A Spanish adaptation of the Western Aphasia Battery (WAB; Kertesz, 1982) and an adaptation of the Pyramids and Palm Trees Test in its word–picture version (Howard & Patterson, 1992) were used to explore semantic processing at the single-word level. In addition, the original versions of both tests were used to assess the aphasia pattern in English. Picture-naming and translation abilities in Spanish and English were further examined using a standardised set of pictures ($N = 100$) from Snodgrass and Vanderwart (1980), as well as a set of verbs ($N = 100$) rated as highly imageable and concrete by five judges. Translation and naming tests were counterbalanced across languages, in two separate sessions. The naming tasks were administered by a monolingual SLP, and the translation tasks were administered by a bilingual SLP. There were five cognates in the verb list (*filmar/to film; galopar/ to gallop; transportar/to transport; robar/rob; aplaudir/to applaud*), and six cognates in the noun list (*barril/barrel; blusa/blouse; botella/bottle; camello/camel; cigarro/cigar; sofa/sofa*).

Results of the pre-therapy assessment. EL's performance on the WAB (Kertesz, 1982) and its translation revealed anomic aphasia in both L1 and L2. EL also presented with minor word-order deficits in the context of sentence and discourse production, as compared to relatively preserved language-comprehension abilities (see Table 1 for results and Table 2 for the percentage of error types). On the Pyramids and Palm Trees Test (Howard & Patterson, 1992), EL scored 52/53 points in both the English version and the Spanish adaptation of the test, thus showing preserved access to semantic information about word targets. With regard to naming, all controls scored 100% in Spanish, regardless of word class, and in English they obtained an average success rate of 96% for nouns and 98% for verbs ($\chi_1^2 = 3.35$, $p = .068$). With translation, all controls scored 100% regardless of language or word class.

In comparison to the controls, EL had impaired word-retrieval abilities across languages, tasks, and grammatical categories (see Figure 1). EL was scored on

TABLE 1
Scores on the WAB oral language tests before therapy

	Spanish	English
I. Spontaneous Speech		
Information content (/10)	8	8
Fluency, grammatical competence (/10)	8	8
II. Auditory Verbal Comprehension		
Yes/No questions (/60)	60	60
Auditory word recognition (/60)	60	60
Sequential commands (/80)	77	71
III. Repetition (/100)	88	84
IV. Naming		
Objects (/60)	37	30
Word fluency (/20)	7	5
Sentence completion (/10)	8	6
Responsive speech (/10)	4	4

TABLE 2
Error types on the WAB naming subtests before therapy

	Spanish		English	
	Anomia	*LS**	*Anomia*	*LS**
Object naming	2	5	4	6
Word fluency	n/a	2	n/a	3
Sentence completion	1	1	2	2
Responsive speech	–	3	1	2
Total number of errors	14		20	
Total per error type	3	11	7	13
% per error type	21%	79%	35%	65%

*LS: Substitution of the target word by its translation equivalent.

accurateness and promptness of response. Thus, promptness is an important measure of functional communication abilities (Frattali, Thompson, Holland, Wohl, & Ferketic, 1995). Correct answers included words named accurately within 5 seconds. Errors were characterised as (a) Language Switching (LS), defined as the substitution of the target word by its translation equivalent; (b) Delayed Naming (DN), a delay of between 5 and 10 seconds before word recall; (c) Anomia, any latency beyond 10 seconds; and (d) Groping Behaviour, the production of word segments that do not lead to target retrieval within 5 seconds.

In Spanish, EL named nouns more easily than verbs ($\chi_1^2 = 9.52$, $p < .01$), while in English his naming of verbs was better than his naming of nouns ($\chi_1^2 = 8.01$, $p < .01$). Moreover access to nouns was significantly more impaired in English than Spanish ($\chi_1^2 = 30.35$, $p < .001$), whereas no such difference across languages was observed for verbs ($\chi_1^2 = 0.084$, *NS*). Translation was better preserved than oral naming across languages. Specifically, translating nouns into English was easier than naming nouns in English ($\chi_1^2 = 10.63$, $p < .001$), and translating verbs into Spanish was easier than naming verbs in Spanish ($\chi_1^2 = 9.58$, $p < .01$). Table 3 shows the percentage of errors in naming and translation. Errors were classified as anomic and language substitutions (LS), defined formally as the substitution of a target by the translation equivalent. Examples of LS of English words when trying to name in Spanish include *table* for *mesa*, *pen* for *lapicera*, and *bee* for *abeja*. Examples of LS to Spanish words when trying to name in English include *auto* for *car*, *fumar* for *smoke*, and *caminar* for *walk*.

Summary of findings and implications at the pre-therapy stage. EL showed anomia and LS on naming tasks. He also showed long latencies, and groping behaviour, particularly on English naming tasks. However, he produced no semantic errors on comprehension tests, and showed preserved oral comprehension abilities. These results, together with his performance on Pyramids and Palm Trees (see Table 1), suggest phonological anomia (Ellis, Franklin, & Crerar, 1994). In addition, as a specific feature of bilingual aphasia, EL could not suppress the non-target language. This resulted in the production of LS in monolingual communicative situations. In most cases, involuntary LS led to communication breakdown. Moreover, attempts to control LS increased anomic signs, such as longer latencies.

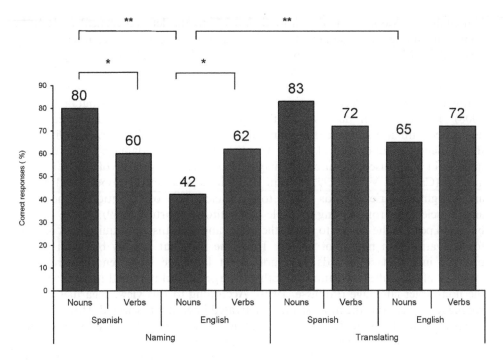

Figure 1. Percentage of correct responses on naming and translation tasks before therapy. $*=p<.01$, $**=p<.001$.

Neurocognitive analysis of EL's language impairment and model-based therapy design

Given EL's profile, our next aim was to develop a theoretically motivated therapy that could be measured against hypotheses derived from neurocognitive models of bilingual language processing. From a neurobiological perspective, EL's language impairment can be described by referring to both neuroimaging data for healthy

TABLE 3
Percentage of correct responses and number of error types with nouns and verbs before therapy

	Naming				Translation			
	Spanish		English		Spanish		English	
	Nouns	Verbs	Nouns	Verbs	Nouns	Verbs	Nouns	Verbs
% Correct	80	60	42	62	83	72	65	72
% Errors	20	40	58	38	17	28	35	28
LS	13	27	32	12	0	0	0	0
DN	–	–	10	12	–	–	–	–
Anomia	7	13	15	8	17	28	35	28
Groping	–	–	1	6	–	–	–	–

LS: Language switching. Substitution of the target word by its translation equivalent.   DN: Delayed naming. Latencies between 5 and 10 seconds, before word access.   Anomia: Latencies beyond 10 seconds.   Groping: The production of word segments not followed by target retrieval within 5 seconds.

bilinguals and lesion data. EL showed damage to the left subcortical perisylvian region, including the caudate nucleus. His language profile was characterised by involuntary LS and anomia in both languages. The role of the basal ganglia in language control has been reported in neuroimaging studies with healthy bilinguals (Abutalebi et al., 2008; Crinion et al., 2006). Recent neuroimaging data suggests that automatic language selection is sustained by the caudate nucleus (Abutalebi et al., 2008). Finally, lesion data shows that damage to the left caudate nucleus is associated with anomic deficits in monolinguals (Cappa & Vallar, 1992). In line with this evidence (Abutalebi et al., 2008; Crinion et al., 2006), damage to the caudate nucleus in EL caused impaired language control, resulting in involuntary LS and anomia (Cappa & Vallar, 1992). From a cognitive perspective, monolingual people are thought to retrieve words thanks to a sufficient flow of activation to the target and its selection from among multiple competitors (Morton, 1969). In the case of bilingual people, the degree to which the target and its translated equivalent compete for activation is a matter of debate. Thus, the fact that healthy bilingual people produce intrusions of words in a non-target language has been interpreted as evidence of a parallel activation of both the target lexical item and its equivalent in the non-target language (Poulisse, 1999). According to this view, regardless of the language spoken, it is the more strongly activated item that is selected. However, this perspective has been challenged by Costa and Caramazza (1999), who showed that raising the activation level of the target's translation not only did not slow target selection but actually speeded it up. Considering the debate (see Costa et al., 2005, for a review), it seems premature to interpret the lesion data from EL as supporting one hypothesis or the other.

LS and word-retrieval deficits can be accounted for elegantly and economically within Green's Activation, Control and Resource Model (Green 1986, 1998a, 1998b). According to this model, successful access to a target word requires sufficient activation flow to access a corresponding lexical node and inhibitory resources to suppress translation equivalents within the bilingual system. Suppression mechanisms may operate either internally, as in translation tasks, or externally, as in the case of conversation conducted in one of the languages spoken (Green, 1986, 1998a, 1998b). Hence, healthy bilingual people can achieve lexical selection of the target with sufficient inhibitory and excitatory resources. The latter activate a target node, while the former suppress the non-target node. According to Green (1986), brain damage can impair the normal selection process and may entail a series of pathological behaviours. In the case of EL, brain damage resulted in insufficient excitatory resources to activate the target, as well as poor inhibitory resources to inhibit the non-target translation. Further, the difference between EL's naming and translation abilities can be accounted for by reference to Green's notion of *schemas*. Schemas are cognitive devices that allow specific language behaviours (i.e., naming, translating, simultaneous interpretation) to be triggered. Thus EL showed better-preserved translation abilities than naming abilities, and this was so across languages and word types. Critically, therefore, EL's performance suggests preservation of the translation schema and impairment of the naming schema. Green's (1986) model also assumes two types of inhibitory mechanisms in the bilingual system: an internal suppression mechanism allowing translation and an external suppression mechanism that allows naming in the target language. EL's translation advantage indicates preserved internal suppression mechanisms but impaired external suppression. In summary, EL's performance provides evidence for possible dissociations between the naming and translation schemas, as well as between internal and external suppression mechanisms, in bilingual people with aphasia.

Our observations provided us with a theoretical basis for selecting therapy methods. Indeed, looking for dissociations such as these may provide cues for custom-tailored therapy in bilingual aphasia. The overall model-based description of EL's pattern resulted in a therapeutic approach that was called *Switch Back Through Translation* (SBTT).

The SBTT approach seeks to exploit preserved internal suppression mechanisms within the translation schema, so as to overcome involuntary switching by translating the word in the non-target language into the target language. This strategy should entail a minimal load on the disrupted external suppression mechanisms, given that EL was not asked to inhibit his English output but to translate it. Thus, whenever involuntary switching occurred, the SLP would implement SBTT. In such cases, she would use a prompt phrase in Spanish to induce translation of the English production into the Spanish target; in this way, a change of schema, from naming (impaired) to translation (preserved) allowed EL to bypass disrupted external suppression mechanisms, and then trigger preserved internal suppression devices, thus facilitating word production. The prompt phrase chosen to induce translation was ... *que quiere decir*... (the English equivalent is "... which means ...") The phrase was pronounced with interrogative prosody, after each LS. Progressively, the SLP replaced the verbal prompt by a hand gesture, and then by a facial gesture (e.g., raising the eyebrows); each time, EL was encouraged to imitate the SLP's gesture while triggering translation. Progressively, EL learnt to use SBTT to cue himself so that he could switch back to Spanish whenever LS occurred.

SBTT was combined with a therapy approach for anomia. Semantic Feature Analysis (Coelho, McHugh, & Boyle, 2000) is a therapy aimed at activating the phonological representations of a target, which is appropriate given EL's anomia pattern. In Semantic Feature Analysis, the SLP asks WH-questions ("What do you do with a pen?" or "Where do you write?"), to increase activation of target semantic features. Boosting the target's semantic representation contributes to activating its phonological representation, and word production. The SLP accepts any answer and shapes it into new WH-questions. If the client is unable to come up with the target after three or four questions, the SLP provides the answer and asks for repetition.

Therapy Stage: Language therapy with SBTT

The primary language of therapy was Spanish; thus, the aim of the therapy was to improve word access in Spanish;[1] all instructions, cueing, and feedback given by the clinician were provided in Spanish only. However, EL was encouraged to express himself in the language that emerged spontaneously. As he was informed of the rationale behind SBTT, he was aware he should not try to inhibit switching to English; instead he was encouraged to follow the cues to switch back to Spanish through translation.

Given that Spanish was the target language of the therapy, only Spanish nouns and verbs were included in the therapy design. Thus, errors with nouns and verbs produced in Spanish naming or in translating to Spanish were assigned to four lists:

---

[1] EL preferred to focus his therapy efforts on Spanish, the language of his environment.

Treated nouns ($N = 20$), Treated verbs ($N = 20$), Control nouns ($N = 15$), and Control verbs ($N = 20$). No cognates were included in the lists.

Stimuli for each session were a series of pictures corresponding to the list of nouns and verbs to be trained. Targets were depicted either in isolation (e.g., a picture of a flower, a picture of someone sleeping) or within graphic stories designed to elicit narrative discourse. Whenever an anomic production occurred, Semantic Feature Analysis was used; whenever LS occurred, SBTT was implemented. In the latter case, EL was progressively encouraged to cue himself with the prompt phrase first, and then gradually with a hand gesture or head movement.

Post-therapy stage: Results following therapy with SBTT

The results on naming and translation tasks are presented in Figure 2. The same error criteria applied in the pre-therapy stage were applied in the post-therapy stage. Further, efficient use of SBTT to overcome LS was considered as a correct response. With regard to naming abilities, the improvement with treated nouns was highly significant (Fisher exact test: $p < .0001$), as was the improvement with treated verbs (Fisher exact test: $p < .0001$). Further, the verbs advantage in English observed before therapy was not present after therapy ($\chi_1^2 = 0.084$, $p = .7$, ns). There was no significant improvement with non-treated Spanish nouns (Fisher exact test: $p = .4$) or verbs (Fisher exact test: $p = .1$). Finally, regarding cross-linguistic effects on the untreated language, the improvement almost reached significance for both nouns ($\chi_1^2 = 3.383$, $p = .062$) and verbs ($\chi_1^2 = 3.31$, $p = .067$).

The results with the translation task into Spanish showed a significant improvement with regard to treated nouns (Fisher exact test: $p < .001$), and treated verbs (Fisher exact test: $p < .001$). With non-treated Spanish words, improvement

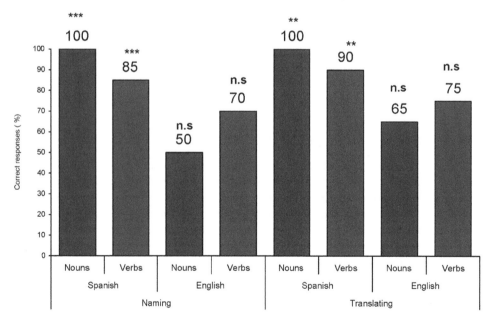

Figure 2. Percentage of correct responses on naming and translation tasks after therapy. $**=p<.001$ (pre- versus post-therapy), $***=p<.0001$ (pre- versus post-therapy).

TABLE 4
Percentage of correct responses and number of error types with nouns and verbs after therapy

	Naming				Translation			
	Spanish		English		Spanish		English	
	Nouns	Verbs	Nouns	Verbs	Nouns	Verbs	Nouns	Verbs
% Correct	100	85	50	70	100	90	65	75
% Errors	0	15	50	30	0	10	35	25
LS	0	0	16	5	0	0	0	0
DN	8	–	–	–	5	–	–	–
Anomia	0	15	44	25	0	10	35	25
Groping	–	–	–	–	–	–	–	–

LS: Language switching. Substitution of the target word by its translation equivalent.   DN: Delayed naming. Latencies between 5 and 10 seconds, before word access.   Anomia: Latencies beyond 10 seconds.   Groping: The production of word segments not followed by target retrieval within 5 seconds.

was significant in verb translation (Fisher exact test: $p < .03$), and almost reached significance with nouns (Fisher exact test: $p = .07$). Regarding cross-linguistic effects of SBTT on the untreated language, no significant effect on translation to English was observed, with either nouns ($\chi_1^2 = 1.135$, $p = .28$, ns) or verbs ($\chi_1^2 = 2.82$, $p = .09$, ns).

Error analysis showed that the number of intrusions decreased considerably across languages, grammatical classes, and tasks (see Table 4). No communication breakdowns were observed in oral naming tasks in Spanish; given that EL would rapidly switch back through translation whenever LS occurred, the communication flow was maintained. Specifically in spontaneous speech, when EL could not overcome anomia, he was able to provide the communication partner with semantic information related to the target (for example: for *bell*, EL said "... you ring it, at school, to go back to the classroom"). Thus, the communication partner would

TABLE 5
Scores on the WAB oral language tests after therapy

	Spanish	English
I. Spontaneous Speech		
Information content (/10)	10	10
Fluency, grammatical competence (/10)	10	8
II. Auditory Verbal Comprehension		
Yes/No questions (/60)	60	60
Auditory word recognition (/60)	60	60
Sequential commands (/80)	81	75
III. Repetition (/100)	96	90
IV. Naming		
Objects (/60)	54	47
Word fluency (/20)	14	9
Sentence completion (/10)	9	7
Responsive Speech (/10)	9	7

TABLE 6
Error types on the WAB naming subtests after therapy

	Spanish		English	
	Anomia	LS*	Anomia	LS*
Object naming	1	1	1	2
Word fluency	N/a	–	N/a	–
Sentence completion	–	1	2	1
Responsive speech	1	–	2	2
Total number of errors	4		10	
Total per error type	2	2	5	5
% per error type	50%	50%	50%	50%

*LS: Language switching: Equivalent word in the non-target language not followed by its translation.

access the word by semantic association or ask EL WH-questions about the target, thereby maintaining the communication flow.

After 3 months of therapy, EL was also retested on the WAB and oral naming and discourse tasks. His results on the WAB are presented in Table 5. EL showed an improvement on naming tasks and a reduction in LS errors across tasks (see Table 6).

DISCUSSION

The purpose of this study was to describe a model-based intervention approach used to improve communication in a bilingual client with chronic aphasia. The client had benefited from language therapy in Spanish in the sub-acute phase following aphasia onset, but had not been able to overcome involuntary LS, and this prevented him from communicating efficiently in everyday life. A pre-therapy assessment showed anomic aphasia in both languages, characterised by impaired LS abilities across naming tasks. An in-depth assessment of naming and translation abilities in both languages showed that translation abilities were better preserved than naming; furthermore, LS errors were by far the greatest source of communication breakdown. Finally, a noun advantage in Spanish and a verb advantage in English were observed in naming.

EL's clinical portrait was interpreted within Green's (1986) ACR model. This allowed us to develop a rationale for therapy with SBTT. Specifically, SBTT made use of preserved internal suppression mechanisms that regulate the translation schema, to induce a switch back to Spanish, whenever the disrupted external device caused inefficient control of L2 in the context of naming in Spanish. SBTT was used together with Semantic Feature Analysis, in the context of language therapy for naming deficits. During therapy both Spanish and English productions were encouraged; there was no inhibition of L2. Instead, EL learnt to use SBTT as a means of switching back to Spanish whenever LS to English occurred. At the beginning of therapy the SLP used a prompt to induce SBTT; gradually EL learnt to cue himself to switch back to Spanish.

The results with SBTT show a significant improvement on naming and translation tasks in Spanish, and no cross-linguistic effects to English. Furthermore, there was a considerable reduction in LS errors across tasks and in both languages. Specifically with naming, SBTT resulted in efficient naming with treated nouns and verbs. With untreated nouns, although all answers given were correct, latency in response was still beyond the cut-off for promptness criteria, with 8 out of 15 untreated items; thus, generalisation to untreated nouns did not reach significance. It is possible that generalisation of SBTT effects to untreated nouns could have reached statistical significance with a larger number of control items. With verbs, anomia was observed with 12 out of 20 untreated items;[2] thus, there was no generalisation to untreated verbs.

Cross-linguistic effects in English did not reach significance. As all unsuccessfully named items before therapy were part of the English word list, the clear lack of generalisation to English cannot be explained by a small number of items and probably relates to the fact that no cognates were included in the therapy list; that is, cross-linguistic effects of therapy may be limited to cognates (Kohnert, 2004).

An unexpected phenomenon emerged with the improvement in naming Spanish verbs. Before therapy, EL showed a noun advantage in Spanish and a verb advantage in English. After therapy, the improvement in Spanish verbs reduced the verb advantage in English (in fact, it was no longer observed). Although an in-depth analysis of this issue is beyond the scope of this paper, it is interesting to note that there are few papers focusing on noun and verb processing following bilingual aphasia (Hernandez, Costa, Sebastian-Gallés, Juncadella, & Reñe, 2007; Kambanaros & van Steenbrugge, 2006; Kremin & De Agostini, 1995; Sasanuma & Park, 1995), and only two report word-category-specific dissociations in naming (Hernandez et al., 2007; Kambanaros & van Steenbrugge, 2006). Hernandez et al. (2007) reported on a highly proficient bilingual woman, suffering from Alzheimer's disease, who showed a verb advantage in naming in L1 and L2. The authors argued that this verb advantage across L1 and L2 indicates that both languages share principles that govern noun–verb representations in the brain. Kambanaros and van Steenbrugge (2006) examined a group of late Greek–English bilinguals with aphasia, and reported cross-linguistic discrepancies in processing of verbs with a noun–name relation. They attributed the opposite pattern of verb processing in Greek (L1) and English (L2) to lower proficiency in L2. In line with this, Guion, Harada, and Clark (2004) argued that late bilingual people, even when highly proficient, may show cross-language differences in word class effects that are not found in early, highly proficient bilingual people or native speakers. It is thus possible that the cross-linguistic discrepancies in verb processing observed with EL reflect the impact of late L2 acquisition. The control participants showed a similar pattern: an advantage with verbs when naming in English. Although not significant, this advantage may reflect a greater facility in processing L2 verbs relative to L2 nouns in late highly proficient bilingual people, as reported in previous studies (Kambanaros & van Steenbrugge, 2006). In EL, the verb advantage was more evident after the stroke but was no longer observed after therapy. However, to provide a definite answer to this question, further assessment would be required.

With regard to translation, SBTT resulted in significant improvement with treated words. Further, there was a generalisation effect to untreated Spanish verbs. Given the improvement in the naming of Spanish verbs previously discussed, and

---

[2] Three anomic errors were observed with treated items as well.

considering that the verb category was significantly more impaired than the noun category before therapy, these results suggest that the effects of SBTT may generalise across tasks within the same language. With untreated nouns, the results were close to reaching significance but did not, because the promptness criterion was not attained with five correctly translated words. It is possible that the small number of nouns (15) in comparison to verbs (20) prevented generalisation effects in translation of nouns from reaching significance. Conversely, SBTT had no impact on translation abilities in the untreated language. In summary, the pattern of results suggests SBTT was an efficient way to treat LS deficits in EL. Improvement was mostly specific to the treated language. However, some generalisation to untreated Spanish items was also observed.

Concluding remarks

Compared to the extensive literature examining therapy aphasia in monolingual speakers, studies on language therapy following bilingual aphasia are rare. It has been assumed that therapy for bilingual aphasia requires the choice of one language and the exclusion of the other, particularly in cases of pathological language switching. This study reports on a model-driven approach to involuntary LS. The model-based interpretation of the clinical phenomena provided a rationale for including both languages in therapy. The therapy, called Switch Back Through Translation, was suited to the strengths and weaknesses of the bilingual client and resulted in improvement. The present study indicates that a theory-driven description of bilingual aphasia, together with a model-based account of dissociations between preserved and disrupted processes in the bilingual language system, can provide cues for efficient intervention in bilingual aphasia. However, further studies are necessary to examine the external validity of SBTT in therapy for bilingual aphasia.

REFERENCES

Abutalebi, J., Annoni, J. M., Zimine, I., Pegna, A. J., Seghier, M. L., & Lee-Jahnke, H. et al. (2008). Language control and lexical comprehension in bilinguals: An event-related fMRI study. *Cerebral Cortex, 18*, 1496–1505.

Ansaldo, A. I., & Marcotte, K. (2007). Language switching in the context of Spanish–English bilingual aphasia. In J. G. Centeno, R. T. Anderson, & L. K. Obler (Eds.), *Communication disorders in Spanish speakers: Theoretical, research, and clinical aspects* (pp. 214–230). Clevedon, UK: Multilingual Matters.

Ansaldo, A. I., Marcotte, K., Scherer, L. C., & Raboyeau, G. (2008). Language therapy and bilingual aphasia: Clinical implications of psycholinguistic and neuroimaging research. *Journal of Neurolinguistics, 21*, 539–557.

Basso, A. (2003). Cognitive rehabilitation. In A. Basso (Ed.), *Aphasia and its therapy*. Oxford, UK: Oxford University Press.

Cappa, S. F., & Vallar, G. (1992). Neurological correlates of recovery in aphasia. *Aphasiology, 6*, 359–372.

Coelho, C., McHugh, R. E., & Boyle, M. (2000). Semantic feature analysis as a treatment for aphasic dysnomia: A replication. *Aphasiology, 14*, 133–142.

Costa, A., & Caramazza, A. (1999). Is lexical selection in bilingual speech production language-specific? Further evidence from Spanish–English and English–Spanish bilinguals. *Bilingualism: Language and Cognition, 2*, 231–244.

Costa, A., Santesteban, M., & Caño, A. (2005). On the facilitatory effects of cognate words in bilingual speech production. *Brain and Language, 94*, 94–103.

Crinion, J., Turner, R., Hanakawa, T., Noppeney, U., Devlin, J. T., & Aso, T. et al. (2006). Language control in the bilingual brain. *Science, 312*, 1537–1540.

Edmonds, L. A., & Kiran, S. (2006). Effect of semantic naming treatment on cross-linguistic generalisation in bilingual aphasia. *Journal of Speech, Language, and Hearing Research, 49*, 729–748.

Ellis, A. W., Franklin, S., & Crerar, A. (1994). Cognitive neuropsychology and the remediation of disorders of spoken language. In M. J. Riddoch & G. W. Humphreys (Eds.), *Cognitive neuropsychology and cognitive rehabilitation* (pp. 287–315). Hove, UK: Lawrence Erlbaum Associates Ltd.

Fabbro, F. (1999). *The neurolinguistics of bilingualism: An introduction*. Hove, UK: Psychology Press.

Frattali, C., Thompson, C., Holland, A., Wohl, C., & Ferketic, M. (1995). *American Speech-Language Learning Association functional assessment of communication skills for adults* (ASHA FAC). Rockville, MD: ASHA.

Galvez, A., & Hinckley, J. J. (2003). Transfer patterns of naming treatment in a case of bilingual aphasia. *Brain and Language, 87*, 173–174.

Green, D. W. (1986). Control, activation, and resource: A framework and a model for the control of speech in bilinguals. *Brain and Language, 27*, 210–223.

Green, D. W. (1998a). Mental control for the bilingual lexico-semantic system. *Bilingualism, 1*, 67–81.

Green, D. W. (1998b). Schemas, tags and inhibition. Reply to commentators. *Bilingualism, 1*, 100–104.

Green, D. W. (2005). The neurocognition of recovery patterns in bilingual aphasics. In J. F. Kroll & A. M. B. De Groot (Eds.), *Handbook of bilingualism: Psycholinguistic approaches* (pp. 516–530). New York: Oxford University Press.

Guion, S., Harada, T., & Clark, J. J. (2004). Early and late Spanish–English bilinguals' acquisition of English word stress patterns. *Bilingualism: Language and Cognition, 7*, 207–226.

Hemphill, R. E. (1976). Polyglot aphasia and polyglot hallucination. In S. Krauss (Ed.), *Encyclopaedic handbook of medical psychology* (pp. 398–400). London: Butterworth.

Hernandez, M., Costa, A., Sebastian-Gallés, N., Juncadella, M., & Reñe, R. (2007). The organisation of nouns and verbs in bilingual speakers: A case of grammatical category-specific deficit. *Journal of Neurolinguistics, 20*, 285–305.

Howard, D., & Patterson, K. (1992). *The Pyramids and Palm Trees Test*. London: Harcourt Assessment.

Kambanaros, M., & van Steenbrugge, W. (2006). Noun and verb processing in Greek–English bilingual individuals with anomic aphasia and the effect of instrumentality and verb–noun relation. *Brain and Language, 97*, 162–177.

Kertesz, A. (1982). *Western aphasia battery*. Orlando, FL: Grune & Stratton.

Kohnert, K. (2004). Cognitive and cognate-based treatments for bilingual aphasia: A case study. *Brain and Language, 91*, 294–302.

Kremin, H., & De Agostini, M. (1995). Impaired and preserved picture naming in two bilingual patients with brain damage. In M. Paradis (Ed.), *Aspects of bilingual aphasia* (pp. 101–110). New York: Elsevier.

Laganaro, M., & Overton Venet, M. (2001). Acquired alexia in multilingual aphasia and computer-assisted treatment in both languages: Issues of generalisation and transfer. *Folia Phoniatrica et Logopaedica, 53*, 135–144.

Lebrun, Y. (1988). Multilinguisme et aphasie. *Revue de Laryngologie, 109*, 299–306.

Marrero, M., Golden, C., & Espe-Pfeifer, P. (2002). Bilingualism, brain injury, and recovery: Implications for understanding the bilingual and for therapy. *Clinical Psychological Review, 22*, 463–478.

Meinzer, M., Obleser, J., Flaisch, T., Eulitz, C., & Rockstroh, B. (2007). Recovery from aphasia as a function of language therapy in an early bilingual patient demonstrated by fMRI. *Neuropsychologia, 45*, 1247–1256.

Morton, J. (1969). Interaction of information in word recognition. *Psychological Review, 76*, 165–178.

Myers-Scotton, C. (2005). *Multiple voices: An introduction to bilingulism*. Blackwell.

Patterson, K. (1994). Reading, writing, and rehabilitation: A reckoning. In M. J. Riddoch & G. W. Humphreys (Eds.), *Cognitive neuropsychology and cognitive rehabilitation* (pp. 425–447). Hove, UK: Lawrence Erlbaum Associates Ltd.

Poulisse, N. (1999). Slips of the tongue. Speech errors in first and second language production. In K. DeBot & T. Heubner (Eds.), *Studies in bilingualism* 20. Amsterdam/Philadelphia: John Benjamins.

Ringbom, H. (2007). *Cross-linguistic similarity in foreign language learning*. Clevedon, UK: Multilingual Matters.

Ruiz, A., & Ansaldo, A. I. (1990). Specific anomia for one language: A cause for language mixing. *Journal of Clinical and Experimental Neuropsychology, 12*, 373–426.

Sasanuma, S., & Park, H. S. (1995). Patterns of language deficits in two Korean–Japanese bilingual aphasic patients: A clinical report. In M. Paradis (Ed.), *Aspects of bilingual aphasia* (pp. 111–123). New York: Elsevier.

Snodgrass, J. G., & Vanderwart, M. (1980). A standardized set of 260 pictures: Norms for name agreement, image agreement, familiarity and visual complexity. *Journal of Experimental Psychology: Human Learning and Memory, 6*, 174–215.

Wertz, R. T. (1999). The role of theory in aphasia: Art or science. In D. Stuss, G. Winocur, & I. H. Robertson (Eds.), *Cognitive neurorehabilitation, part IV* (pp. 265–279). Cambridge, UK: Cambridge University Press.

APHASIOLOGY

Submitting a paper to APHASIOLOGY

Aphasiology is concerned with all aspects of language impairment and related disorders resulting from brain damage. Submissions are encouraged on theoretical, empirical and clinical topics from any disciplinary perspective, and submissions which involve cross disciplinary study are particularly welcome. *Aphasiology* will publish experimental and clinical research papers, reviews, theoretical notes, comments and critiques. Research reports can be group studies, single-case studies or surveys, on psychological, linguistic, medical and social aspects of aphasia. Submissions and ideas for the Review Articles and the Forum are welcome, and interdisciplinary peer commentary is encouraged. *Aphasiology* articles have a maximum limit of 7,500 words. This 7,500 is to include main text only. It excludes title, author's contact details, abstract, references, figures, tables, captions, and footnotes.

Structured Abstracts

Authors submitting papers should note that the journal uses Structured Abstracts. There is good evidence that Structured Abstracts are clearer for readers and facilitate better appropriate indexing and citation of papers.

The essential features of the Structured Abstract are given below. Note in particular that any clinical implications should be clearly stated.

Abstract (Between 150-400 words)

Background: Describe the background to the study.

Aims: State the aims and objectives of the study including any clear research questions or hypotheses.

Methods & Procedures: To include: outline of the methodology and design of experiments; materials employed and subject/participant numbers with basic relevant demographic information; nature of the analyses performed.

Outcomes & Results: Outline the important and relevant results of the analyses.

Conclusions: State the basic conclusions and implications of the study. State, clearly and usefully, if there are implications for management, treatment or service delivery.

Review Abstract

Background: Outline the background to the review.

Aims: State the primary objective of the paper, the reasons behind your critical review and analyses of the literature, and your approach and methods if relevant.

Main Contribution: Give the main outcomes of the paper and results of analyses; and any implications for future research and for management, treatment or service delivery.

Conclusions: State your main conclusions.

All submissions should be made online at *Aphasiology*'s Manuscript Central site (http://mc.manuscriptcentral.com/paph).

Papers are accepted for consideration on condition that you will accept and warrant the following conditions:

1. You will transfer copyright to Psychology Press, should the work be accepted for publication.

2. The work is your original work, and cannot be construed as plagiarising any other published work.

3. You own the copyright in the work.

4. You are empowered by your fellow author(s) to make a submission to this journal, and to make any agreement relating to the work.

5. Your work has not previously been published in the English language.

6. Your work is not under consideration for publication elsewhere, in any form.

7. You have secured the necessary permission in writing from the appropriate authorities for the reproduction in your work of any text, illustration, or other material which is reproduced or derived from a copyrighted source.

8. You have agreed with your fellow author(s) the order of names for publication of the work.

9. You warrant that the work does not include content that is abusive, defamatory, libellous, obscene, fraudulent, or in violation of applicable laws.

If it is found acceptable for publication, you shall retain the right to use the substance of the above work in future works, on condition that you acknowledge its prior publication in the journal, and the publishers Psychology Press.

A complimentary copy of the issue in which your article appears will be sent to the principal or sole author of articles; book reviewers will be sent three copies of the issue free of charge. Offprints may be ordered at a special discount price. An order form will accompany the proof.

Submissions and books for, or offers to, review should be sent to an Editor, address on inside front cover.

Style Guides

Please refer to the following website for the journal style guide, and for more information on our other journals and books: http://www.psypress.com

T - #0027 - 161024 - C0 - 248/168/11 - PB - 9781848727328 - Gloss Lamination